Obstetric Analgesia and Anaesthesia

CURRENT REVIEWS IN OBSTETRICS AND GYNAECOLOGY

OBSTETRICS

Series Editor

Tom Lind MB BS DSc PhD MRCPath MRCOG
MRC Human Reproduction Group, Princess Mary Maternity Hospital, Newcastle upon Tyne

Volumes published

Early Diagnosis of Fetal Defects *D. J. H. Brock*
Early Teenage Pregnancy *J. K. Russell*
Spontaneous Abortion *H. J. Huisjes*
Drugs in Pregnancy *B. Krauer, F. Krauer and F. Hytten*

Volumes in preparation

Coagulation Problem in Pregnancy *E. A. Letsky*
Immunology of Pregnancy *H.Fox and P. Johnson*
Hypertension and Related Problems in Pregnancy *W. A. W. Walters and J. Fidler*
Ultrasound in Obstetrics *W. J. Garrett and P. S. Warren*
Diabetic Pregnancy *M. Brudenell and M. Dodderidge*

GYNAECOLOGY

Series Editors

Albert Singer DPhil PhD FRCOG
Whittington Hospital, London
Joe A. Jordan MD DObst FRCOG
Birmingham Maternity Hospital, Queen Elizabeth Medical Centre, Birmingham

Volumes published

Ovarian Malignancies *M. S. Piver*
Cancer of the Cervix *H. M. Shingleton and J. Orr*

Volumes in preparation

Therapeutic Abortion *A. A. Calder*
Male Infertility *A. M. Jequier*
Gynaecological Premalignant Disease *A. Singer, F. Sharp and J. Jordan*
The Menopause *M. Thom*
Urinary Incontinence *S. L. R. Stanton, L. Cardozo and P. Hilton*
Endometriosis *D. O'Connor*
Endocrine Aspects of Female Infertility *M. Hull*

J. Selwyn Crawford

MB ChB, DA, MD(Ill.), FFARCS, FRCOG

Consultant Anaesthetist, Birmingham Maternity Hospital; Honorary Lecturer in
Obstetric Anaesthesia & Analgesia, University of Birmingham

Obstetric Analgesia and Anaesthesia

Series Editor
TOM LIND

SECOND EDITION

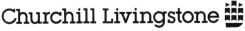

Churchill Livingstone

EDINBURGH LONDON MELBOURNE AND NEW YORK 1984

CHURCHILL LIVINGSTONE
Medical Division of Longman Group Limited

Distributed in the United States of America by Churchill
Livingstone Inc., 19 West 44th Stree, New York, N.Y.
10036, and by associated companies, branches and
representatives throughout the world.

First published 1984

ISBN 0 443 03249 1

British Library Cataloguing in Publication Data
Crawford, J. Selwyn
   Obstetric analgesia and anaesthesia. ——
   2nd ed. —— (Current reviews in obstetrics
   and gynaecology)
   1. Anesthesia in obstetrics
   I. Title   II. Series
   617'9682   RG732

Library of Congress Cataloging in Publication Data
Crawford, J. Selwyn (Jeffrey Selwyn)
   Obstetric analgesia and anaesthesia.
   (Current reviews in obstetrics and gynaecology,
ISSN 0264–5610 ;   )
   Includes index.
   1. Anesthesia in obstetrics. I. Title. II. Series.
[DNLM: 1. Analgesia —— methods. 2. Anesthesia,
Obstetrical —— adverse effects. 3. Anesthesia,
Obstetrical ——
methods. 4. Labor —— drug effects.
W1 CU8093M / WO 450 C8990]
RG732.C69   1984   617'.9682   84–9424

Printed in Great Britain by
Butler & Tanner Ltd, Frome and London

Foreword

When asked to edit this series of short monographs I could think of no-one more suitable to be the first author than Selwyn Crawford. He has made outstanding contributions to the art and science of analgesic and anaesthetic techniques used in obstetric practice and while all of his views may not be accepted by everyone he has made us think. That his approach to the problems of obstetric analgesia and anaesthesia commands wide interest is demonstrated by the fact that the first edition has sold out requiring this second edition only 18 months later. Mindful of the comments made by reviewers and others the author has made changes which further improve upon the quality of the original work. I am confident that this book provides for the needs not only of those reading for higher training examinations but also those requiring a concise, accurate and instructive book to help them undertake these particular aspects of labour ward care.

Newcastle upon Tyne   Tom Lind
1984

Contents

4. Regurgitation and aspiration: causes and management

5. Obstetric and non-obstetric complications affecting anaesthetic practice

The pharmacology of obstetric analgesia and anaesthesia

Factors influencing placental transfer

Although the passage of many substances across the placenta is facilitated by specific transport mechanisms, the transfer of most drugs between mother and fetus does not require such agencies; this is particularly true for those drugs used in the practice of obstetric anaesthesia and analgesia. There are three major physiological determinants of the placental transmission of drugs (Table 1.1).

1. Materno-fetal gradient

Manifestly, the steeper the concentration gradient between maternal and fetal circulations, the greater the amount of drug which must be transmitted in the attempt to achieve equilibrium. However, only rarely, if ever, need consideration be given to the absolute level of drug concentration in the blood of mother or fetus as it reaches the placenta, because that portion of the drug which is bound to plasma protein, or which is held in red cells, is not immediately available for placental transmission. Thus only the unbound drug on each side of the placenta is available for equilibration and the factors which influence both binding and red cell transport are of considerable importance.

Plasma protein concentration. The proportion of systemically-administered drug which is carried through the circulation in the protein-bound form is determined by the concentration of the binding protein and by the acidity of the blood. Under most circumstances, the higher the concentration of the plasma protein involved, the smaller will be the proportion of administered drug

1

which circulates in the unbound form. The carrier protein is usually albumin but globulin binds a significant quantity of some commonly-employed drugs, for example tubocurarine. In obstetric practice this is of special interest because of the characteristic decrease in serum albumin of about 10 grams per litre which occurs by the end of the first trimester. This decrease will, at least theoretically, permit the circulation of a relatively larger proportion of drug in the unbound state, which then becomes available for placental transmission. The tendency will be increased if pre-eclampsia, with its associated fall in serum albumin concentration, develops.

Plasma protein binding. The apparently straightforward relation between protein concentration and binding is rather more complex because the greater the concentration of protein, the smaller is the number of molecules of drug which can be bound by a molecule of protein (Crawford 1969a). This is unlikely significantly to affect the general equation but the availability of binding sites on the protein molecule can be reduced by the adherence of a 'competitive binder'. Thus bilirubin will be displaced from its carrier protein by barbiturates which 'compete' for similar binding sites. An additional factor is the increase during pregnancy (and in women in receipt of an oral contraceptive) of endogenous protein binding inhibitors, including the acute-phase protein alpha$_1$-acid glycoprotein (Levy 1981, Wood & Wood 1981).

Temperature and pH. Although the facility with which a protein molecule binds a drug is temperature dependent, this variant is of no clinical significance; the hydrogen ion concentration of the blood is however of some importance. The degree of protein binding of local anaesthetics is increased by a rise in the pH of the blood (alkalosis), and diminished by acidosis (Tucker & Mather 1975). If small changes in pH within the physiological range cause a clinically significant change in the ability of plasma proteins to bind any particular drug, then factors such as maternal exhaustion or hyperventilation, features common to labour, could become important determinants of the extent of placental transmission.

The discussion has, by inference at least, been concerned with the maternal side of the placental barrier, but similar considerations apply to the fetal side. The continual physiological attempt to achieve equilibrium is influenced only by the unbound fractions of the drug. Once some of the drug has crossed the placenta, part of it will become bound to fetal serum proteins. The ratio between bound and unbound drug in the fetal circulation is however likely to be different from that of maternal blood, for the following three reasons; (i) the concentrations of the various plasma proteins are different, (ii) the pH of fetal blood may be different depending upon clinical circumstances and (iii) the binding capacity of plasma proteins in the fetus is much less than that in the mother, at least in respect of local anaesthetic agents (Ehrnebo et al 1971). This last feature may not be due to a primary difference in binding characteristics of fetal plasma proteins, but rather reflects the influence of other substances within the fetal circulation competing for the same binding sites. It is also worth bearing in mind that in pre-eclampsia, whereas maternal serum albumin concentration falls, that in fetal blood tends to be higher than normal (Studd et al 1972).

Red cell binding. Certain drugs are bound to red cells e.g., local anaesthetic agents and the proportion of drug attached to red cells is unavailable for immediate transmission. The greater the affinity of plasma protein for a drug, the lower will be the proportion bound to red cells, so that for highly protein-bound drugs, such as local anaesthetic agents, the relative binding competition between cells and plasma favours the latter. Some agents have an increased affinity for red cells, e.g. the volatile and gaseous anaesthetics, and for these the higher haematocrit of fetal blood must be remembered.

2. Lipid solubility

The lipid solubility of a drug governs its capacity to traverse the placental barrier because placental cell membranes, in common with all biological membranes, are composed largely of lipoproteins, which are relatively resistant to the passage of water-soluble drugs. There does not appear to be any factor operative in maternal tissues which has the ability to alter the lipid solubility of an administered drug. However, following metabolism, metabolites could be more or less lipid-soluble than the parent drug. Logically, in obstetric anaesthesia and analgesia the choice of a poorly lipid-soluble drug should reduce the amount reaching the fetus; this could however be counter-productive. The blood-brain barrier has properties similar to that of the placenta; hence, to affect the central nervous system and induce sleep or pain relief, a large dose of a poorly lipid-soluble drug will be required and the fetus in turn will receive a proportionately larger amount of that agent.

Highly lipid-soluble drugs should, by definition, be preferentially sequestered in adipose tissues. A placentally-transmitted proportion of a standard dose of drug could thus be less in an obese patient than in a lean person. However, there is an antithetical argument. Blood flow to adipose tissues is a relatively small proportion of cardiac output. The direct effect of drugs having a specific action upon the central nervous system is therefore unlikely to be influenced by the presence or absence of obesity. Further, if the dose of drug to be administered were calculated on the basis of unit mass per kilogram body weight of the patient, this would result, in the case of the obese patient, in a greater than average effect upon the central nervous system.

3. Ionisation

It is reasonable to suppose that the cellular membrane which separates the maternal from the fetal circulation carries a surface charge. Thus any ionised drug will be either repelled by, or held bound to, the surface to which it is presented and only the non-ionised portion will cross the placenta. In general, therefore, poorly-ionised lipid-soluble drugs will cross the placenta with ease while highly-ionised drugs stand little chance of reaching the fetus. However this is a *generalisation* and cannot be taken to imply that highly-ionised drugs will never breach the placental barrier. For example, the muscle relaxant suxamethonium, having been given to a mother in routine dosage, cannot be detected in umbilical vein blood. But if a relatively enormous dose of this drug is injected intravenously as a bolus and umbilical vein blood promptly sampled before a significant hydrolysis of the drug has occurred, then suxamethonium can be detected (Kvisselgaard & Moya 1961). An unusual variant of this situation is when both mother and fetus have an abnormally low level of activity of plasma cholinesterase which is responsible for initiating metabolism of suxamethonium. In such circumstances routine induction of relaxation with a standard dose of this and related drugs could cause consequent neonatal hypotonia (Hoefnagel et al 1979).

The extent to which a drug is ionised when in solution is pH dependant. The pK_a of a drug is the pH value at which the drug is 50 per cent ionised. The environmental temperature in vitro enters into this definition, but is not relevant to in vivo. It follows that the nearer the pK_a is to the physiological range of pH values, the more marked will be the degree of ionisation of the drug resulting from the pH changes which can occur in physically stressed or ill patients. Local anaesthetic agents again provide a good example; the pK_a of procaine is 8.9; at pH 7.0 about 1.2 per cent is unionised which at pH 7.6 increases to only 4.8 per cent. On the other hand, lignocaine, which has a pK_a of 7.9, is 11 per cent unionised at pH 7.0 but at pH 7.6 this proportion increases to *33 per cent* (Ralston & Shnider 1978). Most local anaesthetic agents are weak bases having a pK_a at pH above the physiological range, and thus the more acidic the mother's blood (i.e., the lower the pH) the less will be the proportion of unionised drug available for placental transmission to the fetus. However, the pH value of fetal blood is usually lower than that of maternal arterial blood and the proportion of the drug which is transmitted will be less ionised in the fetal circulation than in the maternal.

Table 1.1 Factors affecting drug transfer between mother and fetus

1. Concentration gradient across the placenta. This is infuenced by:
    a. Degree of protein binding
    b. Blood pH and temperature
    c. Other factors competing for binding sites
    d. Red cell binding capacity

2. Lipid solubility
    a. Similarity between placenta and blood-brain barrier
    b. Loss to fat tissue

3. Degree of ionisation. The effect of pH and pKa

4. Dosage, route of administration and placental circulation

5. Other factors

Three other factors play an important role in determining the extent of placental transfer (Table 1.2).

1. Dosage, route of administration and placental circulation

Several factors govern the concentration achieved at the placental site of an administered dose of drug.

a. Dosage. The greater the mass of drug administered the greater will be the amount available for transfer.

b. Route of administration. For any given mass of administered drug, the more rapidly the entire dose becomes intravascular the greater will be the materno-fetal concentration gradient with the potential for more rapid placental transfer and, under most circumstances, the greater proportion of the dose reaching the fetus. Hence a drug given intravenously as a bolus will not only reach the fetus more rapidly than would be the case if the same dose were given intramuscularly, but in greater amount. The relative delay imposed by the intramuscular route also allows maternal metabolism to dispose of a greater proportion of the drug before it is available for the equilibration process (Crawford 1969b).

Two further points are worth noting regarding the intramuscular route. Some drugs, such as diazepam, are bound to muscle protein to a significant extent, hence a considerable proportion of the drug is sequestered at the site of injection. Secondly, the inclusion of adrenaline reduces the vascularity at the site of injection and therefore the rate at which the drug enters the vascular system. This is particularly relevant to local anaesthetic agents.

c. Interference with blood flow to the placental site. The flow of maternal arterial blood to the placental site is considerably reduced during a uterine contraction. Hence if a bolus of drug is administered intravenously immediately before, or at the start of, a contraction, the highly concentrated 'slug of drug' will have been diminished before it can be presented for transfer across the placenta. This long-held postulate has been supported by the results of at least one report (Haram et al 1978). Conversely, as these investigators pointed out, if the injection were made just before the end of the contraction, then rapid transfer of a greater amount of drug would probably result because of the large influx of arterial blood into the intervillous space.

While uterine artery blood flow can be reduced following compression of the aorta by the gravid uterus, it would be clinically inappropriate to use this manifestation to reduce the transfer of a drug from mother to fetus. Similarly, the fact that local anaesthetic agents used in the paracervical region are likely to cause uterine artery vasoconstriction does not mean that such a technique should be employed as a prophylaxis against placental transmission of the drugs.

2. Molecular size

It is generally accepted that substances with a molecular weight greater than 700 cannot cross the placenta by simple diffusion but none of the agents used for analgesia or anaesthesia even approaches this size.

3. Placental metabolism

Certain drugs are very poorly transmitted because they are effectively metabolised within the placenta e.g., the catecholamines. Noradrenaline will reach the fetus only if a relatively tremendous dose is given to the mother intravenously (Sandler et al 1963), or possibly in the rare clinical circumstance when the mother has a phaeochromocytoma (Morgan et al 1972).

Each of the factors discussed influences the rate and extent of placental transfer but their inter-relations in clinical practice are such that it is impossible to define prospectively, or indeed retrospectively, what proportion of an administered drug will gain entry to the fetus. Broad generalisations are possible: maternal hypoproteinaemia implies that less drug will be bound and more available for placental transmission; maternal alkalosis (related, for example, to hyperventilation) increases the proportion of unionised drug, hence encouraging transfer; fetal acidosis increases ionisation and therefore increases the gradient between fetus and mother; choosing the intravenous route of administration predicates in favour of a relatively greater mass of drug transferring to the fetus.

In many particulars the placental barrier closely resembles the blood-brain barrier. As a rule-of-thumb guide it can be assumed that any drug having a *direct* action upon the central nervous system (c.n.s.) rather than by any effect upon cerebral vasculature, will cross the placenta. A rapidly evoked c.n.s. response will usually be reflected by the equally rapid transmission of a proportion of the drug to the fetus. A prolonged effect upon the c.n.s. would strongly suggest that the drug will be retained in fetal tissues for a considerable length of time.

Table 1.2   Additional factors influencing the placental transfer of drugs

---

1. Concentration at the placental site:
    a. Dose
    b. Route of administration
    c. Placental circulatory dynamics

2. Molecular weight

3. Metabolism within the placenta

Maternal distribution and metabolism of drugs

One of the most important concepts in obstetrics is that the pregnant patient must be regarded as a member of the 'third sex' differing from males and non-pregnant females anatomically, physiologically, emotionally, metabolically and in her capacity to withstand clinical complications such as blood loss. Some of these physiological adaptations may affect drug handling and responsiveness (Table 1.3).

Table 1.3 Factors peculiar to pregnancy (and possibly to pregnancy-like conditions) which influence the distribution, metabolism and responsiveness to drugs

Altered capacity of the liver to metabolise drugs
Increased mass of body fat
Pregnancy specific tissue responsiveness

Liver metabolism. Pregnancy appears to have little effect upon liver function in terms of the usually requested laboratory tests. The increase in alkaline phosphatase results from the placental production of this enzyme, but little is known about the specialised functions of the liver during pregnancy and in particular the metabolism of drugs.

The ability of pregnancy women, as compared with non-pregnant who are not in receipt of an oral contraceptive, to metabolise drugs is a matter of some debate. Although the results of early studies suggest that, for example, pethidine and promazine are less effectively metabolised by the pregnant than by the non-pregnant (Crawford & Rudofsky 1966), subsequent investigators have presented powerful evidence to the contrary (Kuhnert et al 1980, Morrison et al 1982).

It remains a possibility that the dynamics of hepatic enzyme functions are modified by the new hormonal milieu of pregnancy, as is the binding capacity of proteins, as remarked earlier.

Body fat stores. The characteristic increase in body fat of up to four kilograms during pregnancy means that there is a greater capacity for redistribution of lipid-soluble drugs. The relatively low concentration of serum albumin might appear to produce an opposing effect, but the considerable increase of plasma volume results in the total mass of circulating albumin remaining approximately the same in pregnant women as in the non-pregnant.

Tissue responsiveness. There are more specific attributes of pregnancy which infringe upon a mother's responsiveness to drugs. An example of this is the response of the uterine arteries and their tributaries to the application of local anaesthetics. Experiments conducted upon segments of uterine artery obtained from humans (Cibils 1976) and from ewes (Greiss et al 1976) revealed that the application of local anaesthetic solution evoked no response if the donor was non-pregnant or if gestation had not proceeded beyond eight weeks. If, however, the donor had been more than about eight weeks pregnant (in human subjects) the local anaesthetic stimulated a strong contraction of the arterial wall. The concentration required to produce this response was higher than that likely to be achieved in any clinical situation with the exception of paracervical block; but it must now be accepted that drug-induced uterine artery vasospasm is the dominant factor in the association of fetal distress with paracervical block.

Certain inhalational anaesthetics have a direct depressant effect upon the myometrium during pregnancy, although possibly not upon the uterus of the non-pregnant woman. The outstanding examples are chloroform, ether, halothane, and ethrane. Fluroxene and methoryflurane have a similar, although considerably less pronounced, action. The intensity of this action of halothane is such that it can induce myometrial relaxation even in the presence of a high level of concentration of oxytocin. It has been suggested that the effect is not due to a reduction in systemic blood pressure (which each of the four prime agents can induce) but reflects a local increase in the concentration of cyclic adenosine 3^1 5^1 monophosphate (Anderson & Miller 1975). However, it is of some interest to note the close associations which exist between the cardiovascular system and the myometrium.

In general, it can be said that drugs which directly stimulate the myocardium or increase vasomotor tone will enhance myometrial tone and possibly enhance uterine activity e.g., digitalis, quinidine and noradrenaline, while myocardial depressants and vasodilators such as adrenaline, salbutamol, ritodrine and the volatile anaesthetics referred to above will reduce myometrial activity. In an analogous manner ergometrine, which stimulates the myometrium can also induce intense vasoconstriction. There are exceptions however, because prostaglandins and oxytocin which contract the uterus can induce a fall of blood pressure if administered intravenously as a bolus.

9

Points of clinical relevance

Inhalation anaesthesia. Induction of anaesthesia with an inhalational agent is no longer a popular technique in the U.K., intravenous induction agents being much more preferred. However, if an inhalational agent is used, it is advised that the administered level of inspired concentration be lower than that used routinely in the non-pregnant patient. In the spontaneously breathing pregnant patient at term there is a diminished functional residual capacity and an increased minute ventilation. This combination encourages a more rapid achievement of an effective alveolar concentration, and hence a relatively rapid induction of anaesthesia. Furthermore, the spontaneously ventilating pregnant woman requires a lower level of inspired concentration of an inhalational agent to maintain anaesthesia than does a 'matched' non-pregnant woman (Palahniuk et al 1974).

Regional analgesia. An anatomical feature of pregnancy is of considerable importance in regional analgesia. There is considerable distension of the extra-dural veins as pregnancy progresses, with a resultant reduction in the cross-sectional capacity of the extra-dural space. The generally accepted guide is that to achieve the required extent of epidural nerve block, a pregnant patient should be given two-thirds of the dose of local anaesthetic which a non-pregnant woman of similar age and stature would need. The distension of the extra-dural veins is markedly increased if inferior vena caval compression occurs and to a somewhat lesser degree during a uterine contraction. If either of these factors is operative and local anaesthetic is injected, or has been injected, much of the solution remains to be disseminated and the extent of spread could be unexpectedly wide. In the non-pregnant subject the pressure within the epidural space is slightly sub-atmospheric but during pregnancy it is definitely positive, and indeed does not return to the sub-atmospheric status until several hours post-partum (Messih 1981).

Cerebrospinal fluid pressure is unaltered by pregnancy except when the patient is exposed to caval compression or during a uterine contraction. The latter effect is augmented by maternal effort during labour. Under these circumstances the pressure is increased and turbulence may be induced, with the result that local anaesthetic injected intrathecally will be encouraged to spread in a cephalad direction.

Oral administration of drugs. The rate of absorption of orally-administered drugs is unaffected by pregnancy up to the time of onset of the active phase of labour. It was the generally-held belief that depression of gastrointestinal motility and absorptive capacity was a characteristic of active labour. However, most of the studies upon which this view was based were conducted upon patients who had received narcotic analgesics or were in prolonged and exhausting labour. It is now accepted that gastric emptying during labour is not delayed if the patient had not received narcotic agents.

It should nevertheless be noted that the concentration of gastrin in maternal blood has been observed to rise during labour (Athia et al 1982). This suggests that there might be an increase in the gastric residue at this time resulting from an increase in the secretion of water, electrolytes and enzymes into the upper gastrointestinal tract.

Metabolism and distribution of drugs in the fetus and newborn

The fetus

The fetus in utero is not an isolated but otherwise normal little individual; the concentration and characteristics of its serum proteins, the comparative acidosis of its blood and the relatively high value of the fetal haematocrit make it physiologically separate from the mother and these influences have been discussed. Anatomical features specific to the fetus also play a determinant role. Approximately one-seventh of the blood returning via the umbilical vein traverses the ductus venosus, thus bypassing the fetal liver and entering the left atrium directly from the inferior vena cava; it is thus available for presentation to the cerebral circulation and there exists the potential for a considerable transfer of drug from the placenta direct to the fetal brain. Although this might appear to be a rather daunting prospect in respect to drugs which act upon the central nervous system, it is probably of little practical significance in circumstances in which there is a slow, steady transfer of drug across the placenta, as when the drug is administered orally, by inhalation or intramuscularly. The situation possibly becomes more critical if the drug is injected intravenously as a highly concentrated bolus. There is, however, a compensatory influence; the remaining six-sevenths of the umbilical blood flow is directed to the liver and its contents are thus exposed to the actions of hepatic enzymes before being generally distributed to fetal tissues. A drug entering the fetus via the umbilical vein has, therefore, a greater chance of being degraded before general dissemination than does a drug injected intravenously in the adult and, on balance, this may be the dominant influence.

Two further considerations regarding the distribution of drugs within the fetus are worthy of note. There is some evidence to suggest that the fetal blood-brain barrier is more easily penetrable than is the blood-brain barrier of the adult, because of the relatively deficient myelination of fetal neural sheaths (Kupforberg & Way 1963). Secondly, it is only towards the end of gestation that the fetus begins to accumulate a significant mass of adipose tissue. It must therefore be assumed that in mid trimester and the early part of the final trimester, a relatively small proportion of any given lipid-soluble drug can be stored in fetal fat and a higher proportion is thus available to be taken up by more active tissues such as brain and myocardium.

The neonate

The capacity of the neonate to metabolise drugs has been the subject of intensive study and the focus for considerable disagreement over many years. Until it was recognised that the fetus and neonate were not merely miniature adults, it had been tacitly assumed that their metabolising and excretory capacity differed little from that of the adult. Data subsequently became available showing that the fetus at term had not achieved maturity in its capacity to metabolise and excrete certain substances including some drugs. In the view of the present writer, this opinion too is suspect because again the fetal ability is usually compared to that of an adult male or non-pregnant female. As has been stressed, the pregnant patient is physiologically discreet from the non-pregnant adult female, the adaptations being due in large measure to the hormonal status of pregnancy. However, the fetus and to a decreasing extent, the neonate, is exposed to these hormonal influences; when considering processes such as the metabolism of drugs comparison should probably be made between the infant and the *pregnant* subject.

The differing views about the fate of pethidine in the infant afford an excellent example of the current controversy. As has been remarked previously, there is some divergence of opinion about the relative capacity of both the pregnant woman and the neonate to metabolise certain drugs. Major obstacles to the resolution of the problem are the difficulties of assaying the drug and its primary and secondary metabolites in micro-samples of blood and of obtaining complete 24 or 48-hour urinary collections from neonates.

The ultimate experiment would be to administer the drug under review to both mother and infant respectively during the course of the 2–3 weeks following delivery, to observe if the pattern of metabolism and excretion changed as the pregnancy hormonal effects diminished in both, but this is manifestly impracticable on ethical grounds alone. Animal models might seem to be an alternative but it would be unwise to draw conclusions referable to the human from such experiments, because of the well-documented inter-species differences in hepatic enzyme function.

Individual drugs used for analgesia and anaesthesia

Introduction

Consideration of the effects of individual drugs upon the conceptus requires that two distinctions be drawn; the first is whether the reputed effect of a given drug is related to the stage of gestation; the second is whether the effect of a drug is direct or causes some change in the maternal milieu which affects fetal well-being.

Although the prospect that drugs in general taken by the mother during early pregnancy may adversely affect fetal development has been a world-wide concern for several years, very few well-confirmed data have as yet emerged with respect to individual drugs. Analgesics, sedatives and tranquillisers must, for the time being at least, be considered as best avoided during the first 12–16 weeks following conception, if only to reduce maternal concern and avoid possible medico-legal complications. There is no reliable evidence which would support the contention that an anaesthetic agent administered during the first trimester for the relatively brief period of a surgical procedure is detrimental to the subsequent development of the fetus, provided that the mother is not rendered either hypoxic or severely hypotensive (Pederson & Finster 1979). Much heat, but little light, has been engendered in the controversy about the potential dangers of trace quantities of anaesthetic gases. *Abortion and fetal malformation have been associated with the exposure of mothers during pregnancy to trace quantities of*

13

anaesthetic gases and vapours in operating theatres and elsewhere. Most of those who initially supported this association now appear to be softening their attitude; certainly the data available at the present time are not conclusive.

There is little evidence that, subsequent to the first trimester, operative intervention of itself poses a serious threat to the continuance of pregnancy (Brodsky et al 1980). During the first half of pregnancy, intra-abdominal procedures do carry the risk of causing abortion, but this is probably due to the direct stimulation of the uterus during the operation rather than to anaesthetic or analgesic agents. It should be borne in mind that the deliberate induction of abortion has proved to be a difficult task and a surgical procedure performed some distance away from the uterus, whether under the effect of general or regional anaesthesia is unlikely to be harmful. From a clinical viewpoint therefore, any indication for necessary surgery in a pregnant women is not contraindicated because of the potential risk of anaesthetic agents. It is, however, essential that if such a procedure is performed upon a patient who is in the final trimester of pregnancy, great care is taken to ensure that she is not exposed to aorto-caval compression. Such vigilance is required whether the operation is performed in the theatre, the casualty department or the dental surgery.

The list of drugs used to promote anaesthesia, analgesia, sedation, tranquillity and skeletal muscle relaxation is long and increasing. Here we will consider only those in more general use in the U.K. An excellent synopsis, in tabulated form and well referenced, of the effects in the fetus and neonate of maternally administered drugs, will be found in a recent publication (Shnider & Levinson 1979).

Analgesics

Mild analgesic agents

The mild analgesics, such as salicylates, have been suspected of being able to cause congenital defects, but as is the case with so many other drugs and 'pollutants' the association is extremely difficult either to prove or to disprove. Excessive intake of salicylates late in pregnancy can conceivably be of harm to the infant — by displacing bilirubin from albumin or by increasing capillary fragility and reducing platelet adhesiveness — but those doses required would probably be more harmful to the mother.

There is no suggestion that mild analgesics can play an effective role in influencing uterine activity. Salicylates can certainly cross the placental barrier with ease and assessment of their place in obstetric therapy poses an interesting dilemma. On the one hand an increased incidence of stillbirth and of intrauterine growth retardation has been reported as a result of chronic ingestion of aspirin throughout pregnancy. On the other hand, long-term aspirin therapy has been advocated as a means of maintaining efficient intervillous blood-flow in women who appear destined to develop pre-eclampsia.

The opiates

The potential effects of the stronger analgesics upon mother and child are of much greater importance. Although there appears to be no reliable evidence suggesting that the occasional therapeutic dose of a narcotic analgesic during early pregnancy has a deleterious effect upon the infant, the repetitive ingestion of opiates, as in drug addiction, is associated with severe disturbances in the infant. Intra-uterine growth retardation is a characteristic in such cases (Kandall et al 1976) although it is hard to determine how much of this is contributed to by maternal malnourishment and social deprivation. *The neonate of a patient who has sustained her addiction throughout pregnancy can exhibit severe withdrawal symptoms which may persist for a considerable length of time after delivery (Herzlinder et al 1977). However, drug withdrawal during pregnancy can result in premature labour and/or intrauterine death. Complete drug withdrawal should not be attempted during pregnancy. Methadone substitution is the currently advocated form of therapy (Finnegan 1978).*

Note should be taken within this context that the effects upon the infant of maternally-ingested *alcohol* can be even more devastating than those associated with maternal narcotic addiction. The association of a relatively high rate of perinatal mortality and fetal anomalies with maternal alcoholism are now well recognised (Morrison & Maykut 1979), although the level of intake below which these effects are unlikely to result is as yet undefined.

Effect upon labour

Orthodox teaching suggests that powerful depressant drugs can diminish uterine activity and so delay the progress of labour if given in the latent phase; such a view is open to question. It first invites consideration of the definition of the latent phase and obstetricians and anaesthetists have divergent opinions. In unstimulated labour the latent phase is not painful, according to the anaesthetists' definition, and the proposition that powerful analgesics will delay progress is unlikely to have been tested. Contractions which are stimulated or augmented are likely to be painful but they are not depressed by the provision of adequate analgesia.

Uterine activity, whether spontaneous or stimulated, which has reached the active phase is not depressed by narcotic analgesics, or by any other method of pain relief in clinical use. Indeed if pain relief is required but not provided, the consequent maternal distress, metabolic acidosis and eventual exhaustion is likely to cause a reduction in the efficiency of uterine activity (Mark 1961, Maltau & Anderson 1975). In general the better the pain relief the less likely is it that labour will be avoidably prolonged.

Effect upon fetal heart-rate

Diminution or indeed loss of beat-to-beat variability of the fetal heart rate can be caused by a narcotic analgesic. The mechanism involved in this response is not clearly defined; possibly it reflects vagal over-activity or it might be the result of a direct drug effect upon the myocardium. It poses no direct hazard to fetal well-being but the obstetrician must remember to take this drug effect into account when assessing the implications of the fetal heart-rate trace or he may needlessly interfere.

Fetal breathing and movements

Fetal breathing, and possibly fetal movements, are likely to be diminished or even temporarily inhibited by a narcotic analgesic given to the mother, but it seems unlikely that this will be observed during labours conducted in routine clinical practice.

Effect upon the newborn

The effects of maternally-administered narcotic analgesics upon the neonate are well documented. The most important is respiratory depression, due to the direct effect of the narcotic upon the respiratory centre. It is important to bear in mind that this is a purely drug-induced depression, and with absence of other complicating factors, is not accompanied by respiratory acidosis at the time of delivery. The depression can be manifest as hypoventilation of any extent up to and including apnoea. The infant might appear to recover by exhibiting a cry-response to stimulation (preferably slapping the soles of the feet) but its condition will relapse shortly thereafter. Usually poor muscle tone accompanies the respiratory depression, so that the Apgar score is low at one minute. If the appropriate narcotic antagonist is administered (as described in a subsequent chapter) and the infant was not severely asphyxiated at birth, the five-minute Apgar score will be greatly improved. The combined effects of a narcotic and fetal acidosis may cause prolonged post-natal depression; in my experience a low Apgar-minus-colour score at five minutes is especially likely to be recorded for an infant who was delivered with a cord around the neck and whose mother had received pethidine.

General opinion suggests that only if the narcotic analgesic has been given to the mother within six hours of delivery will drug-induced neonatal respiratory depression be seen. This is a convenient guide but by no means an inviolable rule. It is understandable that the longer the time which elapses between administration of the drug to the mother and delivery of the infant, the greater the amount of the drug which will have been metabolised and redistributed and the lower will be the concentration remaining in the mid-brain of the neonate. However, there are innumerable factors which can influence the rate of transfer of a drug from mother to fetus and the dynamics of distribution within fetal tissues. The 'six hour rule' is merely a clinical guideline of the likely outcome. But, clinical experience does teach that if respiratory depression of a neonate is encountered unexpectedly, and the mother has received a narcotic analgesic more than six hours before delivery, a narcotic antagonist should be given and will often effect an improvement in infant status.

Drug-induced neonatal respiratory depression is most likely to occur if a narcotic was given intramuscularly to the mother between two and a half hours and three and a half hours prior to delivery. This has been well documented in a series of cases from which other potentially depressant factors were absent (Shnider & Moya 1964). It is frequently suggested that a narcotic given intramuscularly within half an hour of delivery will not cause neonatal respiratory depression; this proposition is not tenable (Rooth et al 1983). If the drug gives the mother relief from pain (and that, presumably, was the objective), it must have traversed her blood-brain barrier to an appreciable extent, and there is no reason to suppose that it will not also have crossed the placental barrier.

The difference between the various available narcotic analgesics in their respiratory depressant effect upon the neonate is probably of little clinical significance. If equianalgesic doses of the drugs are compared, a similar incidence and severity of depression are likely to be seen, although the results of one study (Way et al 1965) suggested that morphine was a more powerful respiratory depressant than pethidine. It is probable that the feature which distinguishes pethidine from the opiates (morphine, Omnopon and heroin) is that the latter group are much stronger sedatives and general central nervous system depressants. Thus the infant exposed to transplacentally-derived opiate is likely to be less responsive to stimuli, more hypotonic and less active.

Possible long-term effects upon the neonate

Much consideration has recently been given to the longer-term effects of these drugs upon the infant. If a suitable antagonist has not been administered shortly after delivery — and on many occasions the condition of the newly-born infant will not prompt such therapy — evidence of prolonged yet subtle effects may be obtained by the application of neurobehavioural testing. This will show a diminished habituation to stimuli and other discriminatory features of depressed alertness and responsiveness (Hodgkinson & Husain 1982, Wiener et al 1979). However, it must be borne in mind that whilst these tests provide an excellent means of making a fine distinction between the effects of drug administered in clinically acceptable doses to infants who were in other respects healthy, the relevance of the results obtained to the long-term prognosis of infant behavioural responses is highly dubious. *To criticise seriously the prescribing of a drug simply because infants exposed to it exhibit a slightly lower neurobehavioural assessment score than do matched infants exposed to another drug with similar properties would be irresponsible, and serve merely to play into the hands of therapeutic nihilists.* It should be remembered that even a low score based on the relatively crude but widely used five-minute Apgar rating has not been shown to be significantly correlated with the mental outcome and physical development of children who survive beyond the neonatal period.

Local anaesthetics

The use of local anaesthetic agents in obstetric practice has increased following the introduction of epidural analgesia; however they are used by the obstetrician for perineal infiltration, pudendal nerve block and occasionally for paracervical block, and their value and side-effects deserve close consideration.

Toxicity and side-effects in the mother

Although local anaesthetic agents can produce unwanted effects upon the cardiovascular and respiratory systems if given in excessive doses, the dominant clinical concern is with the adverse effects upon the central nervous system. In moderate overdosage these agents can cause drowsiness; this is more likely with lignocaine or mepivacaine than with bupivacaine. *Severe overdosage may cause the patient to convulse or have a series of convulsions.* This is worth bearing in mind if a patient convulses for the first time after delivery and the patient has no other features of eclampsia. Although in the United Kingdom convulsions are the most frequently reported resultants of toxic overdosages, in the United States increasing attention has been directed to the cardiovascular responses (Albright 1982). These consist of bradycardia and hypotension promptly succeeded, in some cases, by cardiac arrest. They appear to be particularly associated with the inadvertent intravenous injection of bupivacaine (as, for example, into an epidural vein) and are strongly reminiscent of the current reports in the U.K. literature of deaths related to the administration of a Bier's block. Moore & Shurlock (1983) have recommended the prompt intravenous administration of adrenaline (0.2–0.3 mg) to correct the myocardial depression in these cases.

It is unrealistic to attempt to define precisely the 'toxic dose' of a local anaesthetic; much will depend upon the route and mode of administration and whether adrenaline is included in the injected mixture. A mass of drug which gains entry into the circulation as a concentrated bolus is more likely to induce cardiovascular or c.n.s. toxicity than is the same mass injected intramuscularly. Similarly, to some extent the more concentrated the solution of drug injected, the lower the mass associated with the likelihood of a toxic response.

The acid-base status and serum protein concentration of maternal blood will also have an influence, as will other maternal medication. The potential toxicity of local anaesthetics is relatively increased if the recipient is acidotic, whether the acidosis is metabolic or respiratory. If the mother has received an anti-convulsant drug, such as diazepam, prior to the injection of local anaesthetic, the concentration of local anaesthetic agent required to trigger a convulsion will be increased, although that required to produce myocardial depression is unlikely to be influenced.

Figures are nevertheless quoted, and the data in Table 1.4 refer to the maximum dose advised at one time.

Table 1.4 The maximum dose of local anaesthetic agent advised at one time

lignocaine without adrenaline	60 ml	0.5 % solution
	30 ml	1.0 % solution
	18 ml	1.5 % solution
	12 ml	2.0 % solution
lignocaine with adrenaline	200 ml	0.5 % solution
	100 ml	1.0 % solution
	75 ml	1.5 % solution
	50 ml	2.0 % solution
mepivacaine (Carbocaine)	80 ml	0.5 % solution
plain	40 ml	1.0 % solution
	20 ml	2.0 % solution
prilocaine (Citanest) plain	20 ml	2.0 % solution
bupivacaine (Marcain) plain	60 ml	0.25% solution
	30 ml	0.5 % solution

Although accumulation of local anaesthetics can occur as a result of repetitive administration, a severe toxic response is unlikely if repeat doses are given only when the analgesic effectiveness of the preceding dose has worn off to an appreciable extent. Such accumulation would usually cause drowsiness, especially those drugs which are markedly protein bound, such as bupivacaine.

Allergic responses to local anaesthetics are extremely rare, but the term is frequently invoked to explain undesired responses which in fact were caused by inappropriate administration of the drug.

Peripheral vascular effects of local anaesthetics, such as hypotension caused by vasomotor block, or uterine artery vasoconstriction, will be discussed in reference to the specific techniques of analgesia (Chapter 2).

The propensity of prilocaine to cause methaemoglobinaemia is worthy of note; this is unlikely to occur in the adult if less than 600 mg of the drug is administered within a relatively short period, but significant conversion of haemoglobin will lead to a reduction in its oxygen-carrying capacity. This is unlikely to cause symptoms if less than half the normal mass of circulating haemoglobin has been converted, but it should be remembered that pregnant women may have a reduced mass if anaemia has developed.

Side effects in the fetus

Local anaesthetics can indirectly affect the fetus by inducing changes in utero-placental circulation, but these factors are discussed in a subsequent chapter. All local anaesthetics can cross the placental barrier and hence affect the fetus directly but the ester-linked agents such as chloroprocaine and procaine are so rapidly hydrolysed by maternal plasma cholinesterase that a very considerable dose would have to be administered for a detectable amount to reach the fetus.

A transient diminution, or occasionally an increase, in beat-to-beat variability, and, much less frequently, late decelerations, have been reported responses to the injection of a local anaesthetic into the mother's epidural space (Lavin et al 1981, Abboud et al 1982). It is suggested that the changes reflect the uptake of the drug by fetal myocardium, but they are acknowledged to be of insignificant import. The only associated hazard is that they are misinterpreted as evidence of fetal compromise, thus initiating a train of unwarranted interference. Severe toxic reactions upon the neonate have been reported following misadventures such as the direct injection of the drug into the fetal scalp and also infiltration of the perineum prior to episiotomy (Kim et al 1979). The response is characterised by convulsions and usually leads to neonatal death.

More subtle effects of local anaesthetics upon the neonate have proved difficult to evaluate in the human. The contention that infant depression in the immediate post-delivery period can be related to transplacentally-derived local anaesthetics has been supported by some investigators and refuted by as many others. Distinctions have also been drawn regarding the identity of the drug used — bupivacaine being generally held to be associated with a lower incidence of sustained, mild depression than lignocaine. The majority of these conclusions have been drawn from the results of neurobehavioural testing of otherwise apparently healthy infants during the hours and days after delivery. It would be tedious to detail all the relevant references and the interested reader can find many of them quoted by Ralston & Shnider (1978) and by Crawford (1984). Suffice it to say that in only a few studies was consideration given to other potential causes of neonatal depression and it would be surprising if the occasional perinate was not found who was particularly susceptible to the depressant action of local anaesthetics, even at a low level present in cord blood.

In most of the reported studies concerned with neurobehavioural assessment of infants the mothers received a continuous lumbar epidural block for labour and delivery. When the local anaesthetic used was either lignocaine or mepivacaine the infants exhibited slight diminution of responsiveness, muscle tone and habituation to stimuli (Scanlon et al 1974), a condition which persisted for more than a week after delivery (Tronick et al 1976). On the other hand, no such deficiencies were found in infants whose mothers had received bupivacaine for epidural analgesia (Scanlon et al 1976, Corke 1977, Hodgkinson et al 1977), but this finding has been challenged (Wiener et al 1979). Any distinction between drugs based solely upon the results of neurobehavioural testing is an interesting and emotive exercise, which has proved useful for quoting to lay audiences in advocacy, or defence, of clinical management; it is probably of very little relevance to the subsequent development of the children concerned. The intriguing possibility that neonatal hyperbilirubinaemia can be caused by bupivacaine administered to the mother requires further investigation (Wood et al 1979).

The pharmacology and clinical effects of local anaesthetics have been succinctly discussed in a monograph by Covino & Vassallo (1976).

Tranquillisers, sedatives and anti-convulsants

The apparently specific term 'tranquilliser' is quite imprecise within the context of clinical practice. Drugs in this category may be used not only as anxiolytics, but as sedatives, anti-convulsants and even employed in obstetric practice as anti-hypertensive agents. In this section drugs will therefore be described in their pharmacological categories.

The phenothiazines and hyoscine

A broad distinction may be drawn between the 'mild' and 'powerful' tranquillisers. The dominant members of the former group in obstetric practice are the phenothiazine derivatives promethazine, promazine and chlorpromazine; the last is a more powerful agent but its value in obstetrics is limited by its propensity for causing biliary stasis and jaundice.

The major virtue of both promethazine and promazine is that neither given in an acceptable clinical dosage causes harm to either mother or infant, but their value as tranquillising agents when given in labour is open to considerable doubt. It could be that the confidence among medical and nursing personnel in this aspect of their action is such that the patient feels better, as in a placebo effect. Thus to advise against the prescribing of these drugs in labour would probably be counter-productive but the informed obstetrician ought to be aware of the true action of the drugs he prescribes. Indeed promethazine has been shown to be an anti-analgesic to some extent, causing diminution of the effectiveness of pethidine if the drugs are given concurrently. Although no convincing evidence has been produced to demonstrate that these phenothiazines have any deleterious effect upon fetal or neonatal well-being, it is known that they cross the placenta rapidly and reach the fetal circulation unchanged.

Hyoscine was the first drug to be demonstrated by chemical analysis to cross the placenta. Although it has sedative and amnesic properties and makes patients feel 'tranquil' its use in the conduct of labour has been virtually abandoned since the end of the era of 'twilight sleep'. Further discussion of this particular drug occurs later in this chapter.

The benzodiazepines

The benzodiazepines can usefully be considered as a group which have sedative and tranquillising properties. The weakest (nitrazepam) will, if given in relatively large dosage, produce similar effects upon mother and infant as will the pharmacologically strongest drug in the group of which the notable members are chlordiazepoxide and diazepam. Each of these, if given to the mother in an increasing dose, will act as a tranquilliser, a sedative or an anti-convulsant. Because only diazepam is generally available for administration intravenously, doctors usually consider it to be an anti-convulsant.

The response to each of the benzodiazepines is markedly dose-dependent and varies with the route of administration. This is particularly true of diazepam and possibly lorazepam although this has not been documented. It has been well demonstrated that if diazepam is injected intramuscularly absorption into the blood tends to be erratic and considerably delayed, possibly because of binding of the drug to muscle protein (Gamble et al 1975, Sturdee 1976). Indeed, in the non-pregnant adult, a dose of diazepam given by mouth is more effective than is the same dose given intramuscularly. *The practice, prevalent in most obstetric units, of administering diazepam intramuscularly rather than intravenously reduces the practical value of the drug by possibly 50 per cent.*

The benzodiazepines cross the placental barrier readily. Diazepam has been identified in fetal scalp capillary blood within one minute following intravenous administration of the drug to the mother (McAllister 1980). *The concentration of chlordiazepoxide* (Decanq et al 1975, Mark & Hamel 1968, Lean et al 1968) *and diazepam* (Hamer & Levy 1980, Gamble et al 1977; *in cord blood at delivery has consistently been found to be higher than that in maternal blood sampled at the same time*, probably reflecting the greater binding power of fetal serum protein. According to one study (McBride et al 1979), this ratio of concentration is reversed in the case of lorazepam. This distinction is apparently a reflection of the capacity of the infant to metabolise and excrete the drugs. Both chlordiazepoxide and diazepam are retained by the neonate for a considerable period, possibly up to a week, after delivery (Cree et al 1973). Furthermore, the primary metabolite of diazepam (dismethyldiazepam) is also pharmacologically active and is excreted at the same slow rate. On the other hand, it appears that the neonate can excrete lorazepam at the same rate as can the mother (McBride et al 1979) and the primary metabolite of this drug is pharmacologically inactive. Yet despite the advantage which this would apparently confer upon the choice of lorazepam, a clinically-directed comparison of the three drugs used as pre-medicants suggested that lorazepam was associated with the highest incidence of prolonged, mild neonatal depression (Crawford 1979).

The benzodiazepines can cause loss of baseline variability of the fetal heart-rate (Yeh et al 1974), a response which may be observed within a few minutes following the intravenous administration of diazepam, and which may persist for more than an hour. It is probably of little significance to the well-being of the infant.

The potential effects of these drugs upon the neonate are closely but not absolutely dose-dependent, and to an extent, are dependent upon the gestational age of the infant at delivery. *The triad of neonatal symptoms is; hypotonia, loss of temperature stability and respiratory depression.*

Hypotonia is the most frequently occurring effect. It can persist for up to 48 hours after delivery but poses no grave threat to neonatal well-being, although the reduced capability to suck and the limp appearance of the infant can alarm the mother and inexperienced attendant staff.

Depression of the temperature-regulating system is potentially dangerous, especially if the infant is pre-term or has low birthweight for gestation, conditions which compromise its capacity to maintain a normal body temperature.

Respiratory depression of a clinically worrying degree is much less frequent, only becoming evident if the mother had received a very large dose of a drug before delivery.

Chlormethiazole, whilst not a benzodiazepine, produces comparable effects to diazepam upon the mother and the new-born. Its main attribute in obstetric practice is its anti-convulsant property.

The barbiturates

The prescribing of barbiturates for sedation is now out of favour in most obstetric departments. The sleep which they produce is on the whole unsatisfactory, they reduce the effectiveness of concurrently-administered analgesics, and, if administered within the period of 12-24 hours before delivery, their depressant action upon the neonate can be markedly prolonged because of its relative inability to metabolise the drug.

Phenobarbitone is an exception; this is still prescribed as an anti-convulsant in the long-term treatment of many epileptics and would be regarded by some as the drug of choice for the pregnant patient. The alternative agents such as primidone and phenytoin sodium have the propensity of causing in the neonate a vitamin K deficiency-like syndrome and have been suggested causal agents for hare-lip and cleft palate. However for the true grand mal epileptic it is unlikely that phenobarbitone alone would be sufficient to prevent attacks.

25

Phenobarbitone is sometimes prescribed for several days prior to the planned delivery of Rhesus-affected infants because it is considered that the drug stimulates hepatic enzyme production and activity, thus helping to limit the post-natal rise in serum bilirubin concentration.

Magnesium sulphate

Magnesium sulphate, for many years the standard anti-convulsant drug used in obstetric practice in the United States, can be discussed here. The term 'anti-convulsant' reflects a mis-interpretation of the role of hypermagnesiumaemia. The raised level of magnesium does not depress cerebral function but causes relaxation of skeletal muscle, peripheral vasodilatation and depression of cardiac rate and conduction (Bradbury 1979). Hypotonia and a reduction of blood pressure are among the initial responses to a therapeutic dose of magnesium sulphate, and increasing doses will, in turn, lead to depression of the deep tendon reflexes, sino-atrial and atrio-ventricular block, respiratory paralysis and eventually cardiac arrest. It has been reported that when magnesium sulphate is given intravenously during labour, a marked decrease of baseline variability in fetal heart-rate occurs within a few minutes (Babaknia & Niebyl 1978), although this has been denied by others (Green et al 1983). The drug crosses the placenta with ease and doubtless contributes to neonatal hypotonia and respiratory depression. However, because the mothers of infants exposed to the drug are almost exclusively suffering from pre-eclampsia, it is difficult to define the contribution made by magnesium sulphate to the neonatal condition.

Drugs given for the conduct of general anaesthesia

Intravenously administered agents

Anti-cholinergic drugs

Many anaesthetists have abandoned the use of either *atropine* or *hyoscine* as pre-medicants because these drugs would have little to offer. Those who continue to employ one or other of the anti-cholinergic agents do so usually as a means of reducing or eliminating the undesirable side-actions of suxamethonium:

stimulation of secretion by the mucus cells of the respiratory endothelium and the salivary glands together with depression of the cardiac conducting systems.

There is probably little to choose between the drugs for these purposes. Hyoscine has been associated with a lower frequency of undesirable maternal hypertension and tachycardia during operation (Shah & Crawford 1969) but the contrast with atropine was not significant. The prospect that hyoscine will induce a phase of amnesia and thus reduce the likelihood that awareness will occur during an operation remains to be proven.

Most anaesthetists who still use these drugs have abandoned the old-fashioned regimen of prescribing them as an intramuscular injection to be given about one hour pre-operatively, and now inject one or other intravenously immediately before induction of anaesthesia. The previous routine offered no advantage and merely provided the patients with a period of disagreeable mouth-dryness and blurred vision. When such an anti-cholinergic agent has been given intravenously, blurred vision may persist for some hours post-operatively and should not be mistaken for a symptom of more ominous import.

Hyoscine, as noted previously, crosses the placenta readily, as does atropine. The latter has been observed to reach the fetal blood within one minute of its intravenous administration to the mother (Kivalo & Saarikoski 1977). It appears to be excreted in neonatal urine largely unmetabolised. Atropine causes fetal tachycardia and at one time the duration of the latent period before this response occurred was advocated as the basis of a test of placental function (Hellman et al 1963) but was abandoned because of unfavourable results (Hellman & Fillisti 1965). Although an 'atropine infusion test' was subsequently described (John 1965) there has been no further reference to its employment. *The use of atropine to reverse fetal bradycardia due to asphyxia would be an unacceptably dangerous procedure*, rather like giving a patient with angina a local anaesthetic to stop the pain and then encouraging him to continue exercising.

Barbiturates

Thiopentone remains the most popular intravenous induction agent. The depth and duration of anaesthesia is to an extent dose-dependant, but because the drug is highly lipid-soluble the duration of its effectiveness is influenced by the amount of well-vascularised fat in the subject's body; poorly-vascularised adipose tissue is of less significance in this respect. Thiopentone is almost universally administered intravenously as a 2.5 per cent solution. When injected at about one millilitre per two seconds it will lead to unconsciousness in 12–20 seconds. If injected more rapidly, a fall of blood pressure is likely to result; because this response is more frequently found when the 5.0 per cent solution is used this strength has, in the main, been abandoned. The duration of unconsciousness which will follow a 'sleep dose' of thiopentone is difficult to assess, depending upon the rapidity of redistribution of the drug from the brain to other tissues and the character of any other drugs which may have been taken by the patient previous to operation. For example other barbiturates, alcohol and opiates make patients 'tolerant' of thiopentone while the stimuli to which the patient is subjected during the period of lightening of anaesthesia will also have an effect. As a rough guide it may be assumed that the normal, healthy pregnant women, unstimulated, will remain anaesthetised for 10–20 minutes following receipt of the customary induction dose (250–300 mg) of thiopentone; but this period will be shortened considerably if a stimulus is applied such as a surgical incision. The resultant problem of 'patient awareness' will be discussed in a subsequent chapter.

The major pharmacologically-associated hazard associated with a thiopentone induction is hypotension. This is of importance in two major clinical circumstances: the patient who is already hypotensive at the start of the procedure and the hypovolaemic patient who, by virtue of peripheral vasoconstriction, is managing to maintain a reasonably normal blood pressure. The loss of vasomotor control caused by thiopentone could lead to a dramatic fall of blood pressure in the latter instance which is not uncommon in obstetric practice. The prospect of such an occurrence must be anticipated and avoided by the use of a much smaller dose of thiopentone and a slower rate of injection.

Like all barbiturates, thiopentone is metabolised in the liver, and any hepatic dysfunction would theoretically reduce the rate of destruction of the drug. In practice the degree of hepatic dysfunction displayed by even the most severely pre-eclamptic patient is rarely sufficient to cause embarrassment in this regard.

In common with all other drugs used to induce anaesthesia, thiopentone being lipid-soluble rapidly reaches the fetus via the placenta. It may be detected in cord blood within less than two minutes following intravenous administration to the mother. The peak concentration in umbilical vein blood is reached in about two or three minutes, the level thereafter falling exponentially. The level in umbilical artery blood rises more slowly and falls parallel to, but at a lower value than, the umbilical vein concentration (Morgan et al 1981). *The fetus is to a considerable extent guarded against the central nervous system depressant action of thiopentone because the major part of the blood flow from the placenta goes first to the fetal liver*; thus a considerable proportion of the received drug is degraded before it has the opportunity of reaching fetal brain. Also, redistribution to non-nervous tissues occurs in the fetus as it does in the mother. As a result it should now be appreciated that the longer the lapse of time between administration of an induction dose of thiopentone to the mother and delivery, the less likely will the infant be depressed by the drug at delivery.

The use of several other intravenous induction agents has been described in the recent literature (Crawford 1984, Shnider & Levinson 1979). *Methohexitone* is rather shorter-acting than thiopentone but appears less likely to cause hypotension. It does seem, however, that any degree of neonatal depression caused is dose dependant (Holdcroft et al 1974). *Ketamine* causes a rise of blood pressure and hence is a drug to be avoided in the treatment of the hypertensive patient. It has also been observed to cause uterine hypertonicity (Galloon 1976, Marx et al 1979). Incoordinate movements and hypertonicity of skeletal muscles are frequently observed during induction with ketamine.

Some disquiet among anaesthetists is caused by the number of reports of sensitivity reactions, including bronchospasm, associated with the bolus use of *althesin* for induction of anaesthesia. *Etomidate* has been considered comparable to thiopentone, but, like ketamine, may cause involuntary movements and hypertonicity. The effects of each of these agents upon the fetus and the ability of the newborn to metabolise and excrete them, has not been as well documented as the effects of thiopentone. However, there is no good reason to believe that spectacular differences will be found, although it has been reported that the incidence of neonatal depression caused by methohexitone (Holdcroft et al 1974) and althesin (Holdcroft et al 1975) is more closely dose-related than is the case with the others. Very recently, althesin has been withdrawn from clinical practice in the UK.

Muscle relaxants

The skeletal muscle relaxants may be considererd pharmacologically in two groups; depolarisers and non-depolarisers. The *depolarisers* trigger stimulation at the neuromuscular junction but induce a much more prolonged refractory phase than does the natural transmitter acetylcholine. The *non-depolarisers* block the action of acetylcholine without initial stimulation.

Depolarising drugs

Suxamethonium, the prime example of a depolarising agent, is hydrolysed by plasma cholinesterase and its duration of action in the normal individual is usually less than five minutes. Subjects with a low level of plasma cholinesterase have a diminished capacity to hydrolyse the relaxant and its activity thus persists for a considerably longer time. Laboratories differ in their estimates of the concentration of cholinesterase in a given sample of blood, but in general it is assumed that if the level found is less than 50 per cent of the range identified as normal, the patient is likely to exhibit a prolonged response to suxamethonium (Whittaker 1980). A low plasma cholinesterase concentration results from genetic factors in roughly one in two thousands subjects. The hereditary transmission is somewhat complicated, involving a silent gene and at least one atypical gene (Whittaker 1980). If a subject demonstrates an unexpectedly prolonged response to suxamethonium and is subsequently shown to have a low level of plasma cholinesterase, efforts should be made to obtain samples of blood from close relatives to establish whether or not they exhibit the same deficiency. Affected subjects should carry a card with the pertinent information noted. Testing of infants should be delayed for six months after delivery, as the deficiency does not manifest itself previous to this in every instance.

The prolonged period of post-operative apnoea, which might occur if suxamethonium has been given in a routine manner to a patient whose cholinesterase deficiency has not been recognised, should not pose a threat to the ultimate well-being of the patient. It means merely that ventilatory support has to be maintained for an extra hour or two following the end of operation to accommodate to the retarded pace of suxamethonium hydrolysis — an embarrassment but not a tragedy.

A reduction of cholinesterase activity in plasma is a characteristic of pregnancy but the extent is not sufficient to influence recovery from the relaxant.

An interesting variant, of which obstetricians should be aware, has recently been described by Evans et al (1980). Plasmapheresis can cause a considerable reduction in the level of cholinesterase activity in the patient's blood; in the pregnant patient whose cholinesterase level is already low, the stage is set for prolonged apnoea to follow the administration of suxamethonium. In the patient with a high Rh antibody titre, referred to in the report, the level of enzyme activity fell progressively after each plasmapheresis because the previous level was not regained by the time the next exchange was performed. Indeed the cholinesterase did not return to a level within the normal range until several weeks after delivery.

The mode of action of suxamethonium causes an initial highly incoordinate 'firing off' at the neuromuscular junctions resulting in a purposeless twitch of the limbs, facial grimacing and a fleeting but sometimes strong spasm of the abdominal muscles. A lower level of response is fibrillary twitching of muscle masses. The manifestation of strong muscle spasm is rarely seen in the pregnant woman (as attested by personal observation of several thousand patients), and this fact has two noteworthy implications. First, intra-abdominal pressure can be considerably raised by spasm of the anterior abdominal wall, with a resultant impetus to the passage of gastric contents up the oesophagus; this is less of a feature in the obstetric patient than many commentators have assumed on the basis of their observations of the non-pregnant.

Second, the severity of the well-known suxamethonium after-pains are to an extent correlated with the intensity of spasm and fasciculations, associated in turn with slight damage to the muscle fibre sheath and release of potassium into the blood. Severe muscle pain in the pregnant or immediately post-partum patient is rare, mild muscle stiffness being reported by only about five per cent (Thind & Bryson 1983). Possibly this is because the progesterone-induced softening of tendons and ligaments characteristic of pregnancy provides sufficient extra elasticity to allow muscle fibre contraction to occur without much local damage. The contrast is so marked that one can almost use it as a test of whether or not the patient was pregnant during the few days previous to operation as, for example, in cases of uterine curettage for vaginal bleeding when an incomplete abortion is suspected.

Suxamethonium, if administered without a preparatory anti-cholinesterase, will stimulate secretion within the respiratory tract but of greater importance, *may cause severe bradycardia*. This response is to be observed most frequently if the relaxant is administered intermittently, especially following the second or third dose, and this technique has been abandoned by many anaesthetists. *Bradycardia is rarely seen as a response to the initial intravenous injection of suxamethonium if atropine or hyoscine has preceded it and is not apparent when the relaxant is given as an intravenous infusion.*

Non-depolarising drugs

These relaxants act by being competitive blockers against acetylcholine at the skeletal neuromuscular junction, thus preventing the muscarinic action of acetylcholine. *Tubocurarine* was the first of these to be introduced into clinical practice and remains the standard agent in the group. Given intravenously its duration of action is of the order of 30–45 minutes, as is that of *pancuronium*, whereas the other popularly-used non-depolarisers have a rather shorter-lasting effect. The activity of tubocurarine is not entirely limited to the skeletal neuromuscular junction. It has been identified as causing a fall of blood pressure, but it is doubtful if this has been of any significance in obstetric practice.

As remarked earlier, the muscle relaxants, being fully ionised, do not cross the placenta when given in clinically acceptable dosage to the mother and pose little or no threat to the fetus. Possible exceptions to this are *alcuronium* (Ho et al 1981) and pancuronium (Duvaldestin et al 1978), which have been found to traverse the placental barrier more readily and are thus better avoided in obstetric practice. It appears that *atracurium* (Frank et al 1983) poses an even greater hazard to the fetus in this respect, although the other recently introduced relaxant, *vercuronium*, given in clinical dosage, reaches the fetus to an insignificant extent (Demetriou 1982). In an early study Crawford (1956) reported that *gallamine* appeared to reach the fetus slightly more readily than did tubocurarine, but *was unlikely to pose a hazard to the infant*. Unfortunately, reviewers and commentators have subsequently asserted, on the basis of this observation, that gallamine is contraindicated in obstetric anaesthetic practice. This is an unjustifiable conclusion but one which has proved difficult to countermand.

Reversal of muscle relaxant effects

It is extremely rare for active measures to be required to counteract the effect of suxamethonium. It is commonly held among anaesthetists that if suxamethonium is given in sufficiently high dosage a 'dual block' can result. The implication is that the relaxant acts initially as a depolariser and subsequently as a non-depolariser, the latter property requiring active reversal. The present writer has personal knowledge of several thousand patients who have received suxamethonium for caesarean section, in doses which have ranged from 300 mg to 1200 mg, and has yet to encounter a single example of a 'dual block'.

A patient who had a total absence of circulating cholinesterase might require an exchange transfusion to encourage hydrolysis of the relaxant but this is a somewhat theoretical situation.

If the activity of a non-depolariser persists beyond the period required for surgery, it may be reversed by the intravenous administration of *neostigmine*. This inhibits the action of acetylcholinesterase, the enzyme responsible for degradation of acetylcholine at the neuromuscular junction and elsewhere. Thus neostigmine permits the accumulation of acetycholine to a local concentration which is sufficient to displace the competitive blocking effect of the non-depolarising relaxant. Unfortunately, neostigmine is non-selective in its activity, and inhibits the metabolism of acetylcholine at all the sites at which the latter is exerting its nicotinic effects, such as in the cardiovascular system, gut, bronchi, eyes and salivary glands. *It is essential therefore that the injection of neostigmine be immediately preceded by one of atropine.* Some anaesthetists give half the atropine before and half with the neostigmine. The usual dose is atropine 1.0 mg and neostigmine 2.5 mg, but the precise dose is tempered to the clinical condition of the patient, to the amount of relaxant received and the time elapsing since the final dose. Usually a single dose of atropine neostigmine is sufficient to achieve permanent reversal of the muscle paralysis and there is no 'hangover' effect, but patients subjected to this treatment must be kept under informed observation for at least one hour. Ideally this would be in a properly-equipped recovery room.

The effect of atropine upon the fetus has already been discussed. There does not appear to be any recorded study of the response of the fetus to transplacentally-derived neostigmine but it would be most unusual for neostigmine to be required in the course of a purely obstetric operation.

In concluding this section one further point must be emphasised; *none of the skeletal muscle relaxants discussed has any direct effect upon uterine tone or activity.*

Inhalational agents

Each of the inhalational agents, if provided in sub-anaesthetic concentration, can be used as an analgesic. Currently in Britain only nitrous oxide (with oxygen as 'Entonox') is employed for this purpose in obstetric practice, trichloroethylene and methoxyflurane having been effectively banned for use by 'unsupervised midwives' in 1983.

There are several ways of categorising inhalational anaesthetics. One is the 'Minimum Alveolar Concentration' (MAC), a concept which was introduced and developed by Eger (1974). The MAC value of an anaesthetic is that which, at one atmosphere, produced immobility in 50 per cent of patients or animals exposed to a strong stimulus; this is usually surgical incision of the skin. Despite its apparent irrelevance to the clinical situation, the MAC value has proved to be closely correlated with the clinical requirements of anaesthesia because the dose-response curve is steep at the point at which the MAC value is reached, and an increase in dose of only 10–15 per cent renders the great majority of patients fully anaesthetised (de Jong & Eger 1975).

The MAC values of commonly-used agents are given in Table 1.5.

Table 1.5 MAC values (in per cent volume per volume) of commonly-used anaesthetic agents

nitrous oxide	101
enflurane	1.68
halothane	0.75
trichlorethylene	0.6
methoxyflurane	0.16

The uptake and distribution of inhalational anaesthetics, the influence upon uptake and distribution of factors such as cardiac output, ventilation-perfusion ratios, ventilatory patterns and lean-to-fat body-mass ratios, have been the subjects of intensive investigation and protracted discourse for many years and while the following generalisations may seem obvious they bear noting:

1. Increasing ventilation leads to an increasing rate of rise of alveolar concentration of the drug.
2. The more soluble the drug the greater will be the increase in the rate of rise of alveolar concentration

The term 'solubility' can have reference to any of a number of conditions, but for our purpose it is sufficient to refer to solubility in blood. The blood-gas partition coefficients (at 37°C) of the agents whose MAC was noted above are given in Table 1.6:

Table 1.6   The blood-gas partition coefficients (at 37°C) of various anaesthetic agents

nitrous oxide	0.47
enflurane	1.9
halothane	2.4
trichloroethylene	9.0
methoxyflurane	13.0

It will be observed that the order of MAC values is the reverse of that of the blood-gas coefficients, which is, of course, no coincidence. From what was said previously, it can also be inferred that, all other things being equal, hyperventilation will be much more effective in increasing the speed of induction of anaesthesia with methoxyflurane than with nitrous oxide.

Changes in cardiac output tend to act in the opposite direction. An increase in cardiac output leads to an increase in the uptake of drug from the alveoli and thus reduces the rate of rise of alveolar concentration. Hence the more soluble the drug the more profound will be the effect of raising cardiac output upon delaying induction of anaesthesia. Conversely, if cardiac output is low, as in the shocked patient or one exposed to inferior vena caval compression, induction with a highly-soluble agent will tend to be facilitated and introduce the hazard of overdosage.

Recovery from inhalational anaesthesia results mainly from excretion via the lungs, although these agents are also metabolised in varying degrees. The rate of recovery is therefore influenced by ventilatory performance (hyperventilation tends to increase the rate), solubility (recovery from poorly-soluble drugs will be more rapid than that from highly-soluble agents) and cardiac output (a high cardiac output is associated with a relatively high rate of transfer of drug from blood to alveoli).

The individual agents have different pharmacological properties additional to those of producing anaesthesia and analgesia.

Halothane has a direct depressant effect upon the circulatory system. It causes a reduction in cardiac output by depressing myocardial contractability. This response is dose-dependent but a significant fall in blood pressure can occur when halothane is given in a concentration appropriate for general surgical rather than obstetric procedures; this will usually be a 1–2 per cent concentration. Halothane also induces peripheral vasodilatation, both venous and arterial, so that perfusion of peripheral tissues in general is well maintained. As remarked earlier, this drug is a powerful myometrial depressant. If uterine relaxation is specifically required, the administration of 2.0 per cent halothane for 90 seconds to the anaesthetised patient will provide it. Recovery of myometrial tone is dependent upon removal of the halothane and cannot be effected by the administration of an oxytocic. *If halothane is used as part of the technique of general anaesthesia for an obstetric procedure in which there is no intent to reduce uterine tone, the administered concentration should not exceed 0.5 volumes per cent.*

Much has been written about the potential ill-effects of halothane upon the liver. The general consensus now appears to be that 'halothane hepatitis' is a rarely-occurring entity, possibly having an immunological component and most likely to be encountered in a patient who receives successive anaesthetics incorporating the drug. The spectre of this occurring in obstetric practice has not been reported, but it is manifestly one to be heeded in gynaecologic practice.

Methoxyflurane also depresses the myocardium but not nearly to the same extent as halothane in equipotent anaesthetic dosage; a hypotensive response to methoxyflurane is infrequent in clinical practice. It has no significant depressant action upon the myometrium and the main concern about this drug has been its effect on the kidney. The nephrotoxicity is not due to methoxyflurane itself but to its degradation products, one of which is oxalic acid and crystals of this chemical may be deposited in the renal tubules. However, it is now doubted that this is the main cause of renal damage and other degradation products, inorganic fluorides, are considered more likely agents. Raised concentrations of these have been identified in both serum and urine. The danger of resultant renal damage is dose-related, the dose being expressed as the factor of inspired concentration times duration of exposure. In order to avoid renal damage, methoxyflurane should be administered at a low concentration for not longer than two hours (Mazze & Cousins 1973) a time limit which should not be reached in the majority of caesarean sections.

Degradation products of methoxyflurane may be detected in cord blood and in neonatal urine but the concentration of fluoride does not give cause for concern.

When methoxyflurane nephrotoxicity was recognised there was concern that the pre-eclamptic patient would be at risk of developing severe renal damage if exposed to even the low dose of the drug used in obstetric practice. This has fortunately proved to be a false alarm.

Trichloroethylene exerts no clinically demonstrative effect upon the cardiovascular system when administered for purposes of either anaesthesia or analgesia. In clinical usage, it is not considered to be hepatotoxic or nephrotoxic, nor does it have a direct effect upon the myometrium.

One of its primary degradation products is trichloroethanol, which is also the active metabolite of chloral hydrate, so that recovery from central nervous depression due to anaesthesia could be delayed by the depression caused by the metabolite. This is of doubtful significance except in cases of prolonged administration.

There appears to have been no reported investigation of the capacity of the neonate to metabolise trichloroethylene. Trichloroethanol will, however, cross the placenta, and if the infant can degrade the anaesthetic agent, and there is no reason for supposing that it cannot, there exists the potential that mild depression of the neonate following administration of trichloroethylene to the mother could be accentuated by the metabolite. *The interaction of trichlorethylene with hot soda lime (the alkaline variety, as used for the absorption of carbon dioxide in closed circuit anaesthesia system) has been recognised for many years, and provides an absolute contra-indication to use of the agent in this system of anaesthesia.* The reaction results in the formation of the toxic compound dichloroacetylene together with a small amount of phosgene, which can cause nerve palsy. Classically this affects the facial nerve and recovery is uncommon.

Nitrous oxide may be considered as an inert agent which has no direct deleterious effect upon the cardiovascular system, liver, kidney, uterus or fetus in clinical obstetric practice. A very prolonged period of exposure to nitrous oxide, amounting to several days, can result in depression of white blood cell maturation with resultant leucopenia but this is largely theoretical. Its major drawback as an independent anaesthetic agent is its relatively low potency. In order to maintain satisfactory surgical anaesthesia it must be administered in an inspired concentration which might imperil oxygenation. Under most conditions of surgical anaesthesia, an inspired oxygen concentration of less than 30 per cent is considered to be highly inadvisable.

Enflurane is one of the more recently introduced volatile agents. It exerts a depressant effect upon the cardiovascular system comparable to that of halothane in equivalent anaesthetic dosage. Its action upon the human pregnant uterus has not been closely investigated but there seems little reason to doubt that, when given in the clinical range of inspired concentration, it will relax the myometrium. Enflurane has not been identified as causing either hepatic or renal damage by direct action, although inorganic fluorides are included among its degradation products.

None of the volatile agents discussed appears to exert any ill-effect upon the perinate other than central nervous system depression. The capacity of the infant to metabolise these drugs is not well documented, but in obstetric analgesia and anaesthesia no evidence has been presented to suggest that these products, whether derived transplacentally or by perinatal metabolism, cause harm to the infant.

Miscellaneous drugs

Some drugs which are frequently used in obstetric practice by both obstetricians and anaesthetists merit brief discussion.

Drugs affecting gastric acidity

Magnesium trisilicate is the main component of the BPC mixture advocated as an antacid preparation. The general use of antacid preparations will be discussed in a later chapter; it is sufficient at this stage to point out that the two-hourly administration of this mixture throughout labour does not cause a significant rise in the level of maternal serum magnesium, and the concentration of serum magnesium in cord blood is barely above the normal range (Aviet & Crawford 1971).

Cimetidine, which is a specific competitive histamine H_2-receptor antagonist, has, as its main action, the inhibition of hydrochloric acid secretion by the gastric mucosa. This drug is currently under review as a prophylaxis against acid-aspiration. When given in clinical dosage either systemically or orally, it has no demonstrable effect upon uterine activity. The placenta appears to offer little resistance to its passage and the drug has been identified in cord blood within five minutes of intravenous administration to the mother (McGowan 1979). There is at present little information regarding the ability of the perinate to metabolise and excrete this drug but infants who have been exposed to it appear to have been clinically unharmed. However, cimetidine does cross the blood-brain barrier and there is a report of its having caused delusional states, agitation and anxiety in elderly subjects who were given several doses of the drug during a 24–36 hour period (Schentag et al 1979). It would seem prudent to discourage the widespread use of the drug in obstetric practice until the results of large, well-controlled and accurately reported trials have testified to its safety.

Ranitidine has an activity similar to that of cimetidine, but of longer duration. Also, according to current reports, it appears not to exert the unwanted side-actions ascribed to cimetidine. Transplacental passage of this drug has been identified, but no harmful effects upon the neonate have been observed to result (McAuley et al 1983).

Although *metoclopramide* is not an antacid, its property of stimulating gastric emptying is occasionally advocated in obstetric anaesthetic practice. Its transfer to the fetus via the placenta has been demonstrated to occur but without resultant ill-effect upon the neonate (Bylsma-Howell et al 1983).

Drugs affecting uterine action

Attention was drawn previously to the intimate relationship which exists pharmacologically between the cardio-vascular system and the myometrium. This becomes significant in several areas of clinical practice. *The drugs which are currently employed as uterine depressants in the attempt to arrest or avert premature labour are also hypotensive agents. It is, therefore, most advisable that if a patient receiving one of these agents comes to require a general anaesthetic or a regional block which involves considerable vasomotor blockade, either (i) assurance be made that the activity of the uterine depressant has worn off, or (ii) the mother's circulation be pre-loaded with at least one litre of crystalloid solution, before induction of anaesthesia or induction of the block.*

The beta adrenergic drug *isoxuprine* gained a modicum of popular usage in the treatment of threatened premature labour. However, it has been reported that neonatal hypoglycaemia, hypocalcaemia, hypotension and ileus, occasionally leading to death, can result if the interval between stopping administration of the drug and delivery of the infant is brief (Brazy & Pupkin 1979). Neither *ritodrine* nor *salbutamol* has been indicted on these counts, but maternal hypotension, tremor, nausea and vomiting are included among the potential side-actions of these drugs.

Ergometrine administered to induce myometrial contractions, will also cause a rise of blood pressure especially in a hypertensive patient. In the awake patient the increase in blood pressure will frequently be accompanied by nausea and vomiting. These responses occur more often after intravenous administration of ergometrine than after intramuscular injection of the drug and in the majority of non-atropinised patients will be accompanied by cardiac irregularities (Baillie 1969). This sequence can cause much chagrin to the anaesthetist as well as distress to the patient particularly if it occurs during the course of a well-conducted regional block for caesarean section. *A truly therapeutic indication to give ergometrine during caesarean section will occur in less than 5 per cent of patients* and the thoughtless 'routine' use of this drug must now be castigated as poor practice. The possibility that ergometrine can cause bronchospasm, especially in the asthmatic patient, has already been mentioned.

Oxytocin provokes a fall of blood pressure and bradycardia when given intravenously as a bolus injection, and in the awake patient nausea and vomiting will frequently accompany these responses. *The effects are very much less likely to occur if the same dose of drug is given in well-diluted form by intravenous infusion*, and in the absence of a compelling reason to the contrary, this must be the preferred method in cases of caesarean section.

Drugs affecting blood pressure

It would be anticipated that agents used in clinical practice to treat hypertension would also exert a depressant effect upon uterine activity. However, this has not been the case when either hydralazine or protoveratrine has been given to pre-eclamptic patients in labour. The effect of these drugs upon the fetus has not been determined. The beta-adrenergic blocking agent, *propranolol*, which may be used as an anti-hypertensive agent, appears to have no significant effect upon uterine activity or tone when given in therapeutic dosage. However, this drug crosses the placenta causing fetal bradycardia and marked hypoglycaemia in the newborn (Habib & McCarthy 1977, Cottrill et al 1977) and it has been suggested as a cause of intra-uterine growth retardation when given earlier in pregnancy (Gladstone et al 1975).

Although it has been demonstrated that *diazoxide* can be passed from mother to fetus, no harm to the neonate appears to result. On the other hand, infants of mothers who have been given *reserpine* have shown serious effects, including lethargy, bradycardia, poor temperature control and a marked degree of nasal congestion which causes considerable respiratory embarrassment.

Drugs affecting urinary output

The use of diuretics in obstetric practice is extremely limited. They are still prescribed for hypertensive mothers in some centres but this practice is not to be recommended; a detailed discussion will be found in a subsequent chapter. The commonly-used diuretic agents undoubtedly traverse the placenta, but there does not appear to be any reported study of mannitol in this regard.

Frusemide administered to the mother has been detected in the blood of the neonate (Beerman et al 1978). It induces a diuresis in the infant causing loss of sodium and potassium via the kidneys (Pecorari et al 1969, Wood et al 1978). Transplacentally-derived thiazide diuretics also deplete the infant of water and electrolytes (Anderson 1970) and have been claimed to cause neonatal thrombocytopenia (Rodriguez et al 1964).

A common form of obstetric mismanagement is to administer to the mother an infusion of dextrose when the requirement is simply for fluid. *Dextrose rapidly traverses the placenta by a process of facilitated diffusion and can be detrimental to fetal and neonatal well-being. Any glucose overload produced may exceed the capacity of the fetus to metabolise the carbohydrate, with the result that accumulation of lactic acid will occur* (Beard & Rivers 1979, Kenepp et al 1980). Such a metabolic acidosis if accompanied by respiratory acidosis and hypoxaemia during labour will result in severe depression of the newborn. A second possibility following the inessential administration of dextrose to the mother is that the induced fetal hyperglycaemia stimulates the fetal pancreatic islet cells to produe insulin so that when the glucose is withdrawn following delivery, neonatal hypoglycaemia results. *Simple fluid replacement for the mother in labour, or preloading before induction of a regional block should be with a crystalloid solution, not with dextrose.*

Anticoagulants

Although *warfarin* and *dicoumarol* are highly-bound to maternal plasma protein, and their presence in the blood of a fetus whose mother has been treated with either of the drugs has not been identified, the consensus of opinion is that they can reach the fetus in a potentially dangerous quantity. On the other hand *heparin*, because of its high molecular weight, traverses the placenta to an insignificant extent.

REFERENCES

Abboud T K, Khoo S S, Miller F, Doan T, Henriksen E M 1982 Maternal, fetal and neonatal responses after epidural anesthesia with bupivacaine, 2 — chloroprocaine or lidocaine. Anesthesia & Analgesia 61: 638

Albright G A 1982 Commentary on: Lalli A F, Amaranath D 1982 A critique on mortality associated with local anaesthetics. Anesthesiology Review 9: 29. In: Obstetric Anesthesia Digest 2: 121

Anderson J B 1970 Effect of diuretics in late pregnancy on the new born infant. Acta Paediatrica Scandinavica 59: 659

Anderson W G, Miller J W 1975 Interaction between Halothane and propanolol on oxytocin-induced uterine contractions. Journal of Pharmacology and Experimental Therapeutics 192: 408

Attia R R, Ebeid A M, Fischer J E, Goudsouzian N G 1982 Maternal, fetal and placental gastrin concentrations. Anaesthesia 37: 18

Aviet T A, Crawford J S 1971 Serum magnesium levels & magnesium trisilicate therapy in labour. British Journal of Anaesthesia 43: 183

Babaknia A, Niebyl J R 1978 Effect of magnesium sulfate on fetal heart-rate baseline variability. Obstetrics and Gynecology 51: 28

Baillie T W 1969 Influence of ergometrine on the initiation of cardiac impulse. Journal of Obstetrics and Gynaecology of the British Commonwealth 76: 34

Baraka A, Haroun S, Bassili M, Abu-Haider G 1975 Response of the newborn to succinylcholine injection to homozygotic atypical mothers. Anesthesiology 43: 115

Beard R W, Rivers R P A 1979 Fetal asphyxia in labour. Lancet 2: 1117

Beerman B, Groschinsky-Grind M, Fahraeus L, Lindstrom B 1978 Placental transfer of frusemide. Clinical Pharmacology & Therapeutics 24: 540

Bradbury M 1979 A concept of the blood-brain barrier. Wiley, Chichester p 385

Brazy J E, Pupkin M J 1979 Effects of maternal isoxuprine administration on pre-term infants. Journal of Pediatrics 94: 444

Brodsky J B, Cohen E N, Brown B W, Wu M L, Whitaker C 1980 Surgery during pregnancy and the fetal outcome. American Journal of Obstetrics & Gynecology 138: 1165

Bylsma-Howell M, Riggs K W, McMorland G H, Rurak D W, Ongley R, McErlane B, Price J D E, Axelson J E 1983 Placental transport of metoclopramide: assessment of maternal and neonatal effects. Canadian Anaesthetists' Society Journal 30: 487

Cibils L A 1976 Response of human uterine arteries to local anesthetics. American Journal of Obstetrics and Gynecology 126: 202

Cooper L V, Stephen G W, Aggett P J A 1977 Elimination of pethidine and bupivacaine in the newborn. Archives of Diseases in Children 52: 638

The pharmacology of obstetric analgesia and anaesthesia

Cottrill C M, McAllister R G, Gettes L, Noonon J A 1977 Propanolol therapy during pregnancy, labor & delivery. Journal of Pediatrics 91: 812

Covino B G, Vassallo H G 1976 Local anesthetics. Greene and Stratton, New York/London

Crawford J S 1969a Drug binding by serum albumin. British Journal of Anaesthesia 41: 543

Crawford J S 1969b Speculation: the sigificance of varying the mode of injection of a drug. British Journal of Anaesthesia 41: 628

Crawford J S 1984 Principles and practice of obstetric anaesthesia, 5th edn. Blackwell, Oxford

Crawford J S 1979 Premedication for elective caesarean section. Anaesthesia 34: 892

Crawford J S, Rudofsky S 1966 Some alterations in the pattern of drug metabolism associated with pregnancy, oral contraceptives and the newly-born. British Journal of Anaesthesia 38: 446

Cree J E, Meyer J, Hailey D M 1973 Diazepam in labour; its metabolism & effect on the clinical condition & thermogenesis of the newborn. British Medical Journal 2: 25

Decanq H E, Bosco J R, Towsend E H 1975 Chordiazepoxide in labor. Journal of Pediatrics 67: 836

De Jong R H, Eger E I 1975 MAC expanded: AD_{50} and AD_{95} values of common inhalation anesthetics in man Anesthesiology 42: 384

Demetriou M, Depoix J P, Diakite B, Fromentin M, Duvaldestin P 1982 Placental transfer of ORG, no. 45 in women undergoing caesarean section. British Journal of Anaesthesia 54: 643

Duvaldestin P, Demetriou M, Henzel D, Desmontis J M 1978 Placental transfer of pancuronium and its pharmacokinetics during caesarean section. Acta anaesthesiologica scandinavica 22: 327

Ehrnebo M, Agurell S, Jalling B et al 1971 Age differences in drug binding by plasma proteins: Studies on human foetuses, neonates and adults. European Journal of Clinical Pharmacology 3: 189

Eger E I 1974 Anesthetic uptake & action. Williams & Wilkins, Baltimore

Evans R T, MacDonald R, Robinson A 1980 Suxamethonium apnoea associated with plasmaphoresis. Anaesthesia 35: 198

Finnegan L P 1978 Management of pregnant drug-dependant women. Annals of the New York Academy of Sciences 311: 135

Frank M, Flynn J P, Hughes R 1983 Atracurium in obstetric anaesthesia. British Journal of Anaesthesia 55: 1135

Galloon S 1976 Ketamine for obstetric delivery. Anesthesiology 44: 522

Gamble J A S, Dundee J W, Assaf R A E 1975 Plasma diazepam levels after single dose oral & intramuscular injection. Anaesthesia 30: 164

Gamble J A S, Moore J, Lamki H, Howard P J 1977 A study of diazepam levels in mother & infant. British Journal of Obstetrics and Gynaecology 84: 588

Gladstone G R, Hordof A, Gersony W M 1975 Propanolol administration during pregnancy: effects on fetus. Journal of Pediatrics 85: 962

Green K W, Kay T C, Coen R, Rasnik R 1983 The effects of maternally administered magnesium sulfate on the infant. American Journal of Obstetrics & Gynecology 146: 29

Greiss F C, Still J G, Anderson S G 1976 Effects of local anesthetic agents on the uterine vasculature & myometrium. American Journal of Obstetrics and Gynecology 124: 889

Habib A, McCarthy J S 1977 Effects on the neonate of propanolol administered during pregnancy. Journal of Pediatrics 91: 808

Hamer C, Levy G 1980 Serum protein binding of drugs and bilirubin in newborn infants and their mothers. Clinical Pharmacology and Therapeutics 28: 58

Haram K, Bakke O M, Johannessen K H, Lund T 1978 Transplacental passage of diazepam during labor; influence of uterine contractions. Clinical Pharmacology and Therapeutics 24: 590

Hellman L M, Morton G W, Tolles W E, Fillisti L P 1963 Computer analysis of the atropine test for placental function. American Journal of Obstetrics and Gynecology 85: 610

Hellman L M, Fillisti L P 1965 Analysis of the atropine test for placental transfer in gravidas with toxemia and diabetes. American Journal of Obstetrics and Gynecology 91: 787

Herzlinder R A, Kandall S R, Vaughan H G 1977 Neonatal seizures associated with narcotic withdrawal. Journal of Pediatrics 91: 638

Ho P C, Stephens I D, Triggs E J 1981 Caesarean section and placental transfer of alcuronium. Anaesthesia and Intensive Care 9: 113

Hodgkinson R, Husain F J 1982 Duration of effect of maternally administered meperidine on neonatal neurobehaviour. Anesthesiology 56: 51

Hoefnagel D, Harris A, Kin T H 1979 Transient respiratory depression of the newborn. American Journal of Diseases of Children 133: 825

Holdcroft A, Robinson M J, Gordon H, Whitwam J G 1974 Comparison of effects of two induction doses of methohexitone on infants delivered by elective Caesarean Section. British Medical Journal 2: 472

Holdcroft A, Morgan M, Gordon H, Whitwam J G, White Y 1975 Althesin as an induction agent for caesarean section. British Journal of Anaesthesia 47: 1213

John A H 1965 Placental transfer of atropine and the effect on foetal herat-rate. British Journal of Anaesthesia 37: 57

Kandall S R, Albin S, Lowinson J et al 1976 Differential effects of maternal heroin and methadone use on birth weight. Pediatrics 58: 681

Kenepp N B, Sheeley W C, Kumar S, Gutsche B B, Gabbe S, Deliviora-Papadopoulos M 1980 Correspondence: Effects on newborn of hydration with glucose in patients undergoing Caesarean section with regional anaesthesia. Lancet 1: 645

Kim W Y, Pomerance J J, Miller A A 1979 Lidocaine intoxication in a newborn following local anesthesia for episiotomy. Pediatrics 64: 643

Kavalo I, Saarikoski S 1977 Placental transmission of atropine at full-term pregnancy. British Journal of Anaesthesia 49: 1017

Kuhnert B R, Kuhnert P M, Tu A-S, Lin D C K, Foltz R L 1979 Meperidine and normeperidine levels following meperidine administration during labor. I. Mother. American Journal of Obstetrics and Gynecology 133: 904

Kuhnert B R, Kuhnert P M, Tu A-S, Lin D C K 1979 Meperidine and normeperidine levels following meperidine administration during labor II Fetus and neonate. American Journal of Obstetrics and Gynecology 133: 909

Kuhnert B R, Kuhnert P M, Prochasaka A L, Sokol R J 1980 Meperidine distribution in mother, neonate and non pregnant females. Clinical Pharmacology & Therapeutics 27: 486

Kupforberg J H, Way E L 1963 Pharmacologic basis for the increased sensitivity of the newborn rat to morphine. Journal of Pharmacology and Experimental Therapeutics 141: 105

Kvisselgaard N, Moya F 1961 Investigation of placental thresholds to succinylcholine. Anesthesiology 22: 7

Lavin J P, Samuels S V, Miodovnik M, Holroyde J, Loon M, Joyce T 1981 Effects of bupivacaine and chloroprocaine as local anesthetic for epidural anesthesia on fetal heart rate monitoring patterns. American Journal of Obstetrics & Gynecology 141: 717

Lean T H, Ratnam S S, Sivasamboo R 1968 Use of chlordiazepoxide in patients with severe pregnancy toxaemia. Journal of Obstetrics and Gynaecology of the British Commonwealth 75: 853

Levy G 1981 Pharmacokinetics of fetal and neonatal exposure to drugs. Obstetrics & Gynecology 58: suppl. 9S

McAllister C B 1980 Placental transfer and neonatal effects of diazepam when administered to women just before delivery. British Journal of Anaesthesia 52: 423

McAuley D M, Moore J, McCaughey W, Donnelly B D, Dundee J W 1983 Ranitidine as an antacid before elective caesarean section. Anaesthesia 38: 108

Maltau J M, Anderson H T 1975 Epidural analgesia as an alternative to caesarean section in the treatment of prolonged exhaustive labour. Acta Anaesthesiologica Scandinavica 19: 348

Mark R F 1961 Dependance of uterine muscle contractions on pH, with reference to prolonged labour. Journal of Obstetrics and Gynaecology of the British Commonwealth 68: 584

Mark P M, Hamel J 1968 Librium for patients in labor. Obstetrics and Gynecology 32: 188

Marx G F, Hwang H S, Chandra P 1979 Postpartum uterine pressures with different doses of ketamine. Anesthesiology 50: 163

Mazze R I, Cousins M J 1973 Methoxyflurane nephrotoxicity: a study of dose-response in man. Journal of the American Medical Association 255: 1611

McBride R J, Dundee J W, Moore J, Toner W, Howard P J 1979 A study of the plasma concentrations of lorazepam in mothers and neonates. British Journal of Anaesthesia 61: 971

McGowan W A W 1979 Safety of cimetidine in obstetric patients. Journal of the Royal Society of Medicine 72: 902

Messih M N A 1981 Epidural space pressures in the lumbar region during pregnancy. Anaesthesia 36: 775

Moore D C, Scurlock J E 1983 Possible role of epinephrine in prevention or correction of myocardial depression associated with bupivacaine. Anesthesia & Analgesia 62: 450

Morgan C D, Sandler M, Panigel M 1972 Placentral transfer of catecholamines in vitro and in vivo. American Journal of Obstetrics and Gynecology 122: 1068

Morgan D J, Blackman G L, Paull J D, Wolf L J 1981 Pharmacokinetics and plasma binding of thiopental II. Studies at cesarean section. Anesthesiology 54: 474

Morrison A B, Maykut M O 1979 Potential adverse effects of maternal alcohol ingestion on the developing fetus and their sequelae in the infant and child. Canadian Medical Association Journal 120: 826

Morrison J C, Todd E L, Lipshitz J, Anderson G D, Schneider J M, Dilts P V 1982 Meperidine metabolism in the parturient. Obstetrics & Gynecology 59: 359

Nimmo W S, Wilson J, Prescott L F 1975 Narcotic analgesics & delayed gastric emptying in labour. Lancet 1: 890

Owens D, Zeitlin G L 1975 Hypoventilation in a newborn following administration of succinylcholine to the mother. Current Researches in Anesthesia and Analgesia 54: 38

Palahniuk R J, Shnider S M, Eger E I 1974 Pregnancy decreases the requirements for inhaled anesthetic agents. Anesthesiology 41: 82

Pecorari D, Ragni N, Autera C 1969 Effects on the newborn of the injection of frusemide to the mother during labour. Acta Biomedica 40: 89

Pederson H, Finster M 1979 Anesthetic risk in the pregnant surgical patient. Anesthesiology 51: 439

Rodriguez S V, Leikin S L, Hiller M C 1964 Neonatal thrombocytopenia associated with antepartum administration of thiazide drugs. New England Journal of Medicine 270: 881

Rooth G, Lysikiewicz A, Huch R, Huch A 1983 Some effects of maternal pethidine administration on the newborn. British Journal of Obstetrics & Gynaecology 90: 28

Sandler M, Ruthvan C R J, Contractor S F, Wood C, Booth R T, Pinkerton J H M 1963 Transmission of noradrenaline across the human placenta. Nature 197: 598

Schentag J J, Callreri G, Rose J Q, Cerra F B, DeGlopper E, Bernhard W 1979 Pharmacokinetic & clinical studies in patients with cimetidine-associated mental confusion. Lancet 1: 177

Shah J, Crawford J S 1969 Cardiovascular responses observed in obstetric patients premedicated with either atropine or hyoscine. British Journal of Anaesthesia 41: 557

Shnider S M, Moya F 1964 Effects of meperidine on the newborn infant. American Journal of Obstetrics and Gynecology 89: 1009

Shnider S M, Levinson G 1979 Anesthesia for obstetrics. Williams & Wilkins, Baltimore/London

Studd J W W, Shaw R W, Bailey D E 1972 Maternal and fetal serum protein concentrations in normal pregnancy and pregnancy complicated by proteinuric pre-eclampsia. American Journal of Obstetrics & Gynecology 114: 582

Sturdee D W 1976 Diazepam: routes of administration & rate of absorption. British Journal of Anaesthesia 48: 1091

Thind G S, Bryson T H L 1983 Single dose suxamethonium and muscle pain in pregnancy. British Journal of Anaesthesia 55: 743

Tucker G T, Mather L E 1975 Pharmacokinetics of local anaesthetic agents. British Journal of Anaesthesia 47: 213

Way W L, Costley E C, Way E L 1965 Respiratory sensitivity of the newborn infant to meperidine and morphine. Clinical Pharmacology and Therapeutics 6: 454

Whittaker M 1980 Plasma cholinesterase variants & the anaesthetist. Anaesthesia 35: 174

Wood B, Culley P, Roginski C, Powell J, Waterhouse J 1979 Factors affecting neonatal jaundice. Archives of Disease in Childhood 54: 111

Wood M W, Wood A J J 1981 Changes in plasma drug binding and alpha$_1$-acid glycoprotein in mother and newborn infant. Clinical Pharmacology & Therapeutics 29: 522

Wood W-C R, Dupont C, Collinge J, Aranda J 1978 Effects of frusemide in the newborn. Clinical Pharmacology and Therapeutics 23: 266

Yeh S Y, Paul R H, Cordero L, Hon E H 1974 A study of diazepam during labor. Obstetrics & Gynecology 43: 363

Zargham I, Leviss S R, Marx G F 1974 Uterine pressures during fluroxene anesthesia. Current Researches in Anesthesia and Analgesia 53: 568

2

Relief from pain and anxiety in labour

The anxiety of labour

The major fault of the early adherents of Grantly Dick-Read's 'Natural Childbirth' and similar movements lay in their inability to accept that 'normal' labour could require the use of pain-relieving agents. Many of the patients who, having experienced as much pain as they could bear, asked for pharmacological relief, were subsequently rendered distraught because of feeling a failure in the 'natural' sense. It is essential that any system of preparation for childbirth includes (i) an acknowledgement that pain can be an unavoidable feature of labour in many women, (ii) an assurance that if and when the need arises relief will be provided and (iii) an exposition (and where appropriate a demonstration) of the range of techniques of analgesia available in the Obstetric Unit. An account of the latter should include a sensibly modulated reference to both the advantages and disadvantages to mother and baby of the individual methods.

It is unfortunate that currently, one extreme wing of the psychoprophylaxis school has disregarded the lessons which should have been learned from the Dick-Read history. Even more unfortunately, not only are these exponents claiming to provide comfort in labour, but also are suggesting that adherence to their method will ensure that the child, at delivery and during subsequent development, will be of a quality superior to that which would otherwise have been the case. The appeal of such promises is obviously great, especially to those sections of the community already in sympathy with anti-science, anti-technology, and 'return-to-nature' movements. There is, however, no reliable evidence that the methods advocated by Lamaze and Leboyer confer any notable advantage to either mother or infant. On the contrary, the few controlled series which have been reported have served to demonstrate that there is virtually no significant difference between study group patients and controls in respect to labour, delivery, condition of the infant at delivery, subsequent development of the child and mother-child relationship (Scott & Rose 1976, Hughey et al 1978, Nelson et al 1980). The group of control subjects must be composed of patients who have been given preparatory advice and who do not enter upon labour in a state of extreme anxiety. It has been demonstrated (Morishima et al 1978) that fear and apprehension can lead to a rise in maternal blood pressure, an increase in uterine activity, fetal bradycardia and intra-uterine asphyxia. *It is frequently forgotten that the pharmacological management of pain-relief during labour must be supported by measures to provide relief from anxiety as well.*

Melzak and his colleagues, during the past two decades, have established international pre-eminence in respect to their studies of the physiology and assessment of pain. After spending 15 years studying various categories of pain they came to investigate the pain of labour. In a compelling report (Melzak et al 1981) they presented evidence that labour pain was the most severe they had ever assessed. Of equal interest was their observation that, among women who had received a well-modulated and sympathetic preparation for childbirth, the mean pain score during labour was some 30 per cent lower than the mean score among those who entered upon labour without good preparation — although it was still higher than the mean score associated with any other type of pain. Among the subjects observed by these workers were six who had received antenatal preparation from an enthusiastic exponent of the Lamaze technique.

The pain of labour

The pain of labour is multifactorial in origin (Table 2.1). The major component results from contraction of the myometrial fibres; this is possibly ischaemic pain, although the evidence in support of such a contention is inconclusive. Pain originating from the uterus is transmitted to the spinal cord via the sensory fibres of the T11 and T12 nerve roots, with some overflow (possibly 'reverberation') via T10 and L1. *The upper and lower uterine segments do not have sensory nerve supplies of differing root*

Table 2.1 Pain associated with labour

Site of origin	Characteristic stimulus	Neural involvement	Localisation
Uterus	contraction — ?ischaemic ?plus acute stretch	sympathetic outflow, root values T11/12 spreading to T10 & L1	referred to distribution anterior rami (X2) of somatic roots: upper abdominal wall anteriorly down to groin; inner aspects upper thighs
Peri-uterine tissues, mainly posterior	pressure — either with contractions or persistent. Usually associated with fetal malposition or unusual conformation of sacrum	somatic roots of lumbo-sacral plexus	typically, distribution of posterior low & mid-back; also back of thighs
Lower birth canal	distension of vagina and perineum in second-stage	somatic roots S2/3/4	accurate to site of stimulus (i.e., not referred)
Bladder	over-distension; can be persistent or felt only during contraction	sympathetic (T11–?L2) via hypogastric plexus, parasympathetic (S2/3/4)	usually suprapubic only; rarely referred to distribution of somatic sacral roots
Myometrium & uterine visceral peritoneum	abruption; scar dehiscence	T10–L1	accurate to surface marking of site of pathology

values; the cervic is served by sensory nerves of the same root value as is the fundus. There is, however, one difference which is worth noting: most sensory nerve fibres reach the uterus via the base of the broad ligament, but some fibres travel via the ovarian plexus, from where they are distributed mainy to the fundus. The importance of the anatomical route is that a paracervical block will not affect the passage of impulses which pass along these latter fibres and hence will not relieve all uterine sensation.

Additional pain synchronous with contractions may occur as a result of pressure of the uterus against surrounding structures, particularly those within the posterior wall of the pelvis such as muscle fascia and possibly the nerve trunks of the lumbo-sacral plexuses. Under such circumstances pain will be appreciated in the lower part of the back (posterior roots of the lumbar outflow) and possibly in the upper thighs. Severe sustained pressure such as is typically associated with a persistent occipito-posterior position, or with a 'flat sacrum', is likely to cause pain which persists even between contractions. If the forward movement of the upper part of the uterus during a contraction is resisted by a tense anterior abdominal wall, this too may lead to discomfort or pain, which is likely to be felt suprapubically.

Subsequent to full dilatation of the cervix and during delivery there can be additional sources of pain perhaps due to distortion of the pelvic floor and distension of the vagina; such pain impulses are transmitted by sensory nerves of root value S2, 3 and 4.

Two other potential sources of pain in labour are worth noting; first, the urinary bladder receives its sensory nerve supply via S2, 3 and 4, and if it is allowed to become over-distended, pain will be experienced in the perineum and in the immediate suprapubic region. Second, complications arising in the substance of the myometrium can be strikingly painful. Frequently a patient who has had a small placental abruption, or whose uterine scar is in the process of rupturing, will be able to indicate the site of pathology with reasonable accuracy.

The urge to 'bear down' is a reflex response; it is initiated by distension of the pelvic floor, the sensory arc of the reflex being served by the nerves of root value S2, 3 and 4. The motor side of the reflex involves the muscles of the anterior abdominal wall, the diaphragm and the glottis. The pelvic floor muscles are in the main supplied by motor fibres of root value S2, 3 and 4; their tone and contraction during the second-stage of labour aid in manoeuvring the presenting part on its journey, but may increase the associated

Table 2.2 Items contributing to relief from pain & anxiety during labour

Educational

Ante-natal information, advice & reassurance
Relaxation classes
Structured lectures & demonstrations

Environmental

Sympathetic & attentive staff (medical & nursing)
Pleasant surroundings
Attendance of husband

Pharmacologic

A. Analgesia

   1. Self administered inhalational (Entonox). In active first-stage start inhalation at onset of contraction; subsequent to full cervical dilatation anticipate contraction by 30 seconds. 30–40% fully satisfied; 30% fail.
   2. Narcotic analgesia. Pethidine 100 mg (occasionally 150 mg) intramuscularly. Possibly repeat after 3–4 hours. Less favoured alternatives, morphine 10 mg; Omnopon 15 mg; pentazocine 60 mg; self-administered intravenous pethidine.
   3. Regional analgesia
      a. Paracervical: now infrequently used, and then only if no evidence suggestive of fetus 'at risk'.
      b. Spinal: inappropriate early in active phase first-stage; good if late first-stage or in second-stage & instrumental delivery anticipated.
      c. Extra-dural: (i) caudal — disadvantages are that anatomical variations of sacral hiatus make initiation difficult or impossible in 5%; large volume of local anaesthetic required; sacral roots inevitably blocked first.
         (ii) lumbar — bupivacaine 0.25–0.5%. Range of indications increased & of contraindications diminished with increasing experience in the delivery suite. 85% fully satisfied; 3% fail.

B. Relief from anxiety
Promazine (50 mg i.m.) tranquillising activity not very impressive, but affords no harm to mother or infant.
Diazepam (5 mg, occasionally 10 mg, preferably intravenously well-diluted). Powerful c.n.s. depressant; potential effects on neonate include hypotonia, temperature instability and respiratory depression.

pain because of the increased muscle resistance rather than pelvic floor relaxation.

There is no evidence that the pain of labour affords any advantage to either mother or child. Phylogenetically it possibly provided a warning that delivery was imminent, but it is doubtful if it plays a significant role in this regard in *Homo sapiens*. Culturally, a virtue has been made out of this embarrassing phylogenetic remnant, to the extent that acceptance of pain has been held to represent some sort of maternal triumph over adversity. Whatever the merits of such a concept, it has become apparent during recent years that pain, if permitted to become more than a little obtrusive, prompts a series of metabolic responses in the mother which, in some instances, are reflected in the fetus. These include a progressive increase in metabolic acidosis (Pearson & Davies 1973, Pearson & Davies 1974), an increase in the concentration of plasma cortisol and a fall in plasma oestriol levels (Maltau et al 1979), a rise in the concentration of plasma beta endorphins (Abboud et al 1983) and an incease in the level of concentration of circulating catacholamines (Jones & Greiss 1982, Shnider et al 1983). Total abolition of pain prevents these changes from occurring but does not interfere with the orderly progress of labour.

Techniques of analgesia

Systemically-administered drugs

Narcotics. There are few significant differences in potency between the narcotic analgesics generally available for clinical use. Pethidine remains the standard drug, as it has since the mid-1930s, being preferred to morphia, heroin and Omnopon because these are much more powerful soporifics. Pethidine is predominantly an analgesic and should not be referred to as a 'sedative'. It is now customary for a labouring patient to receive one dose of pethidine, usually 100 mg given intramuscularly; rarely in modern obstetric practice would more than two such doses be required. When given by intramuscular injection the onset of action of this drug will not become appreciable for 10–15 minutes and patients should be warned that two or three contractions subsequent to the injection will cause as much pain as did the previous ones; it usually provides a reasonable degree of analgesia for the next three hours. Its potential side-effects have been detailed previously; they include dizziness, a degree of dissociation, drowsiness, nausea, vomiting and occasionally a fall in blood pressure. It does not seem to affect adversely the progress of labour but its efficiency as an analgesic is open to question. One of the few well-controlled studies designed to assess the value of pethidine (Beazley et al 1967), revealed that fewer than one-quarter of the patients so treated had a pain-free labour, whereas 40 per cent reported that they had not experienced any relief. A technique whereby incremental doses of a dilute solution of pethidine are administered intravenously by a patient-activated system using either an infusion (Scott 1970) or a syringe pump (Evans et al 1976) offers the prospect of a higher quality of analgesia. Such devices incorporate safety features designed to avoid any possibility of over-dosage but there is no indication yet that these systems are becoming popular on a national scale. The apparatus is particularly valuable in the care of mothers with a coagulation defect, for whom an epidural is contraindicated and intramuscular injections inadvisable. It is salutory to record that, in our experience, mothers who are provided with this apparatus will be found, not infrequently, to have self-administered 300–400 mg pethidine during a labour of average duration: evidence surely of the relative inadequacy of our established advocated regimens.

It is important to appreciate that the Central Midwives Board does not stipulate or restrict the choice of narcotic analgesic used by 'unsupervised midwives', a phrase which usually denotes midwives in domiciliary practice. The confines within which such midwives must work are at the discretion of Medical Officer of Health or any doctor of analogous status.

Two other narcotic analgesics should be mentioned, pentazocine and butorphanol.

Pentazocine was introduced with a flourish some years ago as the first no-addicting narcotic; *it has subsequently been identified as a drug of addiction,* although considerably less so than pethidine or the opiates. *It was considered initially that, dose for dose, it was at least twice as powerful as pethidine in its analgesic property; this opinion too, has been modified.* In current practice pentazocine is given intramuscularly in a dose of 50–60 mg, and its duration of action is briefer than that of pethidine; the degree of neonatal respiratory depression following a single dose of pentazocine is indistinguishable from that caused by pethidine. However if multiple doses of either drug have been given to mothers, the infants appear to be more severely affected following the use of pethidine. The conclusion drawn was that whereas the neonatal response to pethidine was cumulative, with pentazocine the response reaches a maximum at the maternal dose of about 60 mg per 70 kg (Refstad & Lindback 1980). The hallucinogenic property of pentazocine has mitigated against its use in many centres.

Butorphanol in a dose of 1–2 mg intramuscularly has been compared with 80 mg of pethidine and found to provide equally satisfactory analgesia; the same incidence of maternal side-effects and the same incidence and degree of neonatal depression have been reported however (Maduska & Hajghassemali 1978).

53

Narcotic antagonists. The major concern about using pethidine during labour is the prospect of neonatal respiratory depression. The tenuous relation between the time of administration of the drug and delivery of the infant with regard to such depression has been discussed previously. Narcotic-induced respiratory depression can be reversed by the administration of a narcotic antagonist. Three such agents have been, or are, in clinical use.

Nalorphine does not require much discussion as its use in obstetric and neonatal practice has been abandoned. If given in a dose greater than required to offset the respiratory depression caused by a narcotic analgesic, the respiratory depression may be worsened. The popularity of levallorphan is also waning because it too carries the potential of causing respiratory depression if it is over-titrated, although the safety margin is very much greater than with nalorphine. *Naloxone* on the other hand, is reputed to be a pure narcotic antagonist although reports are emerging which suggest that it has analeptic properties.

It is neither necessary nor advisable to administer either of these two antagonists to the mother in the expectation of averting neonatal respiratory depression. The medical and nursing staff should be aware that an infant may be at risk of respiratory depression and be prepared to treat it promptly; to treat the fetus blindly, when it may be quite unnecessary to do so, is poor medical practice. Furthermore, both levallorphan and, more particularly, naloxone reduce the analgesic property of pethidine.

If levallorphan is used it should be injected intramuscularly in a dose of 0.25 mg to an infant who is 2.5 kg or more or 0.125 mg to an infant of less than 2.5 kg; the injection site is then massaged. If the respiratory depression had indeed been due mainly to the narcotic, the infant will begin to cry vigorously in 90 seconds.

It was originally suggested that naloxone should be given intravenously in a dose of 40 micrograms (Evans et al 1976). Unfortunately the duration of activity of naloxone is appreciably shorter than that of pethidine and the action of the antagonist may wear off allowing the pethidine effect to re-appear in an infant who might not be under close observation. *The current advice is that naloxone should be given by intramuscular injection in a standard dose of 200 micrograms* (Wiener et al 1977). This can entail some delay in the effective response to the antagonist and if the imposition of such a delay, which might be a matter of one or two minutes, is considered to be inadvisable, 40 micrograms of naloxone should be given intravenously as well as the 200 micrograms intramuscularly. This drug does appear to prevent or considerably diminish the longer-term depressant effects of pethidine upon the neonate (Wiener et al 1977, Wiener et al 1979, Brice et al 1979).

Tranquillising agents. Even if relief from pain is complete, maternal anxiety can still be disturbing. If it has not proved possible to calm the mother's fears by sympathetic reassurance and encouragement, a tranquilliser should be given both to reduce maternal distress and to prevent the associated fetal distress (Morishima et al 1978). Currently the choice lies predominantly between two drugs, *promazine* and *diazepam*. The former is a relatively weak anxiolytic but has the outstanding attribute of not posing a threat to perinatal well-being. It is usually given intramuscularly in a dose of 50 mg, which can be repeated but will rarely be needed more than twice in the course of a labour. Diazepam is a much more powerful central nervous depressant; the effects upon mother and infant and the arguments in favour of preferring to inject it intravenously rather than intramuscularly have been detailed in Chapter 1. When diazepam is prescribed simply as an anxiolytic and not as part of a regimen in the treatment of a pre-eclamptic patient, the preferable dose is 5 mg, although a severely agitated patient especially one of large stature, might require 10 mg to attain an adequate response. Very rarely should the need arise to give more than one dose of diazepam during labour of those patients in whom pregnancy has been uncomplicated. The effects of diazepam upon the neonate cannot be reversed pharmacologically.

Intermittent inhalational analgesia

In 1983 the Central Midwives Board withdrew approval for the use of trichloroethylene by unsupervised midwives, and effectively ensured the abandonment of methoxyflurane. Thus only nitrous oxide remains for discussion in this context.

For almost three decades *nitrous oxide* was provided as a 50:50 mixture with air by means of the Minnitt's 'gas and air' apparatus. Although this proved to be popular and apparently free from maternal or perinatal complications the fact that the inhaled mixture contained only 10 per cent oxygen led to increasing unease. Indeed on occasion even less than 10 per cent oxygen was given because of faults in apparatuses in clinical use. In the early 1960s the CMB withdrew its permission for 'unsupervised midwives' to use Minnitt's apparatus, and recognised Entonox in its place.

The introduction of the Entonox system was the result of the almost single-handed dedication and hard work of Tunstall (1961). The system consists of a cylinder, a simple reducing valve and a demand valve with appropriate tubing and mask. The cylinder contains a premixed mixture of nitrous oxide and oxygen in a ratio of 50:50 a tolerance of one per cent being permitted. The physical state of the pre-mixed gases remains somewhat of a puzzle but its outstanding attribute is that the composition remains constant throughout the time taken for the cylinder to empty. There is one important exception to this statement: *if the contents of the cylinder are allowed to cool below minus 6°C the constituent gases will begin to separate. Nitrous oxide is more dense than oxygen, and if separation occurs and reconstitution of the mixture is not undertaken, the first gas to issue will be predominantly oxygen and subsequently the gas will be almost pure nitrous oxide.* Temperatures below freezing point are not uncommon in Britain, and cylinders could well be exposed to them during overnight transport on lorries or when stored in hospital grounds. The pre-mixed mixture can be reconstituted by rewarming the cylinder and then inverting it three times. This procedure is feasible with the small (500 l) cylinders destined for domiciliary use, but it is not easily performed with the much larger cylinders generally used in hospital practice. The rules which are to be followed with regard to these are based upon the advice of an MRC Committee which considered the problem (Cole et al 1970).

a. On receipt of the cylinder by the hospital, the cylinder should be date-marked, and before use, stored in a horizontal position for 24 hours in an area maintained at a temperature above 10°C, but not exceeding 45°C;

b. During delivery from the storage area to the final destination point in the hospital, the cylinder must not be exposed to freezing temperature for more than 10 minutes.

Satisfactory analgesia will be obtained by self-administration of Entonox if the correct technique is employed. It is unfortunate but true that although self-administered intermittent inhalational analgesia remains the most widely-used method in obstetric practive in the U.K., woefully little attention is paid to assuring that the niceties of the technique, which are necessary to its successful application, are followed. *Obstetricians and midwives alike display an inexcusable ignorance in this field.*

In the active phase of the first-stage of labour — and in the latent phase of stimulated labour — although a contraction lasts for almost one minute, the first 20–30 seconds of the contraction are usually not painful. The reason is easy to understand: the pain of a uterine contraction is of ischaemic origin, and the delay reflects the time taken for the products of local metabolism to reach a level of concentration sufficient to initiate painful stimuli. It takes this same period, approximately 20–30 seconds of deep panting using the Entonox apparatus to achieve a sufficient concentration of nitrous oxide in the appropriate c.n.s. centres to provide for analgesia. Thus the technique required to achieve success in the first-stage is for the mother to start self-administration at the very beginning of the contraction, and to continue the administration until the contraction has ended. *Delaying the start of administration until pain is felt is a guarantee that analgesia will not be obtained, and is the major reason for discontent with this method of pain relief.*

Two refinements are worthy of note. During the relaxation phase of a contraction arterialised blood regains entry to the myometrium, relieving the ischaemia. Thus the mother might find it unnecessary to continue taking Entonox throughout the period of a contraction. Secondly, when the interval between contractions is very brief there will possibly be insufficient time for complete 'wash out' of metabolic degradation products to be effected, so that pain will reappear with less than the usual delay after the start of a contraction. In this situation the provision of a low baseline concentration of continuously inspired Entonox could be of value (Arthurs & Rosen 1981).

It is equally important to appreciate that the situation changes subsequent to full cervical dilatation. The reason is that pain from distension of the pelvic floor and lower birth canal is not ischaemia but is due simply to stretching of the tissues which form these structures. Now the contraction, which will again last for about a minute, is likely to be painful from its onset, and the mother will have the added urge to 'bear down'. There is thus no useful warning to indicate when self-administration should start. Reliance must be placed upon the fact that at this time the contractions tend to occur quite regularly, the interval between being reasonably consistent. Ante-natally, the mother must be taught to anicipate the contraction by beginning to pant from the apparatus 30 seconds before the contraction is due to begin. When the contraction starts, the bearing down reflex is stimulated and the mother will begin to push. It is unlikely that she will be able to do this for more than 10–11 seconds each time, and she will then pant from the apparatus, then bear-down again, and so forth until the end of the contraction. Failure to anticipate the start of a contraction will invite a distressing and painful second-stage.

Many consider that, to reduce perineal trauma, the mother should be discouraged from bearing-down during the time the head is crossing the perineum. Encouraging the mother to pant hard from her inhalational apparatus before and throughout a contraction is helpful in subduing the bearing-down reflex during this phase.

Entonox may be self-administered intermittently throughout a labour of any length. There is no deterrent to the provision of analgesia with both the inhalational agent and a narcotic analgesic during the same labour, although such a practice does tend to increase the likelihood that the mother will lose self-control and hence look back upon her labour with dissatisfaction. The effectiveness of Entonox in preventing the pain of labour is of approximately the same order as that of pethidine; 23 per cent total success; 40 per cent total failure (Beazley et al 1967).

Nitrous oxide is rapidly and completely eliminated via the lungs after it has been inhaled during a contraction, and thus the ventilatory effort required to achieve a satisfactory dose can be considered as remaining the same throughout labour.

Provision of inhalational analgesia is strongly indicated in the delivery suite during surgical induction of labour and the first formal vaginal examination of a patient in early labour. A considerable proportion of mothers who are subjected to these procedures find them to be extremely uncomfortable or painful. The results of one study (Caseby 1974) suggested that almost one-quarter of the patients who have an artificial rupture of the membranes consider it to be painful — in many instances it is the most painful episode during their stay in the delivery suite. There is no reasonable excuse for allowing this barbarity to persist. By encouraging the mother to pant from her inhalational analgesic apparatus for a couple of minutes before the start of the procedure, and to continue to do so until completion of the procedure, pain and discomfort will be averted without affording any danger to either mother or fetus.

Finally, mention should be made of a recently-introduced modification of the traditional apparatus; the substitution of a mouth-piece for the face-mask (Dolan & Rosen 1975). Many people have a horror of anaesthetic masks and the mouth-piece has proved to be a most acceptable alternative in several obstetric centres. The CMB, however has not yet approved its use by 'unsupervised midwives'.

Regional analgesia for labour

The techniques of regional analgesia will be discussed in ascending order of current clinical interest and practice.

i. Spinal block

The institution of spinal analgesia early in the active phase of the first-stage of labour has not gained general acceptance in the U.K. Although 'continuous spinal block' maintained by intermittent injection into the cerebrospinal fluid via a cannula is practised in one or two reputable centres in the world, many clinicians avoid this technique because of its potential complications. Usually spinal analgesia is a single shot procedure and the duration of its effectiveness depends to an extent upon the choice of drug employed. This will be discussed in detail in a subsequent chapter, but it may be noted here that in current clinical practice the duration of satisfactory analgesia would be unlikely to exceed four hours. The provision of a spinal block is, therefore, reserved for the mother whose labour has either reached the end of the first-stage, or has entered the second-stage, and who appears likely to require an operative vaginal delivery. Further discussion is reserved for a later chapter.

ii. Paravertebral block

This consists of the deposition of local anaesthetic in the region of the roots of the nerves involved in the pain of the first-stage (T10–12, L1) as they traverse the paravertebral region. By repetitive redirecting of the needle, the block may be executed via a single site of entry through the skin on each side. Although the technique was employed occasionally in obstetric practice several years ago, it demanded considerable expertise and only provided relief during the first-stage. These features discouraged its more widespread application.

59

iii. Lumbar sympathetic block

This procedure is intended to block the sensory nerve fibres from the myometrium as they are carried within the lumbar portion of the sympathetic chains. According to a recent study (Meguiar & Wheeler 1978) 10 ml of 0.5 per cent bupivacaine solution containing adrenaline injected in the vicinity of each lumbar sympathetic chain is relatively successful in relieving the pain of a uterine contraction. The procedure is more difficult to conduct than a lumbar epidural block and more painful for the patient, but the investigators suggested that it might have an occasional place in the care of a patient in whom entry into the extra-dural space proved to be impossible.

iv. Paracervical block

Paracervical block is accomplished by inserting an appropriately sheathed needle with a blunt-ended guard 1–2 cm through the mucosa of each lateral fornix of the vagina and, after performing an aspiration test, depositing 5–10 ml of local anaesthetic solution in each paracervical region. The objective is to block impulses travelling in the sensory nerves which supply the uterus. The reported incidence of achieving successful analgesia is of the order of 80 per cent (Belfrage et al 1983). The duration of effectiveness, using 0.25 per cent bupivacaine, averages a little over 1 hour (Belfrage et al 1983, Nesheim et al 1983). To some extent, the degree of effectiveness must depend upon the vagaries of the precise location of the sensory nerves within the base of the broad ligament. Another determinant is the extent to which uterine sensation is subserved by nerves which travel via the ovarian plexuses, and hence will not be effected by the procedure.

Paracervical block gained widespread popularity in the 1960s, despite the fact that it is almost invariably used as an intermittent or single-shot technique and only provides relief from the pain of the first-stage of labour; possibly its appeal lay in the fact that its accomplishment lay within the natural province of the obstetrician. However, doubts soon began to be raised about the safety of the method in respect to the fetus.

A high incidence of fetal bradycardia is associated with paracervical block, usually becoming evident within a few minutes of its initiation and associated with a fall in fetal scalp blood pH and oxygen tension (Baxi et al 1979). This evidence of fetal asphyxia characteristically persists for about half an hour and although recovery usually takes place, there have been isolated reports of fetal deaths which appear to have resulted directly from the regional block. Elucidation of the specific factors which caused the fetal asphyxia was the focus of much investigation and debate for several years; a favoured suggestion at one time was that the fetal myocardium was depressed by the direct effect of local anaesthetic carried to the placental site after absorption through the wall of the uterine arteries. However, what appears to be the true explanation was provided by Cibilis (1976) and Greiss et al (1976) who demonstrated that the application of an anaesthetic solution to a segment of uterine artery obtained from a pregnant human or animal, in a concentration comparable to that likely to be attained in the production of a paracervical block, leads to a marked degree of vasoconstriction. Fetal asphyxia after a paracervical block may therefore be caused by a diminution in utero-placental blood flow resulting from uterine artery constriction. The local anaesthetic agent used is apparently of little significance in this regard. Even the rapidly-hydrolysed chloro-procaine has been implicated (Weiss et al 1977).

Paracervical block continues to be used in several centres, notably in the United States and Scandinavia, but with considerable circumspection. *Even the more inveterate users of the technique advocate that it must not be employed in any case in which there is presumptive evidence of fetal compromise.*

v. Extra-dural block

The extra-dural space extends from the foramen magnum to the sacrococcygeal membrane. Internally it is bound by the dura mater, externally it is bound by the bony vertebral canal which is discontinuous. Between the vertebal bodies, anterior to the extra-dural space, are the intervertebral discs. The posterior longitudinal ligament, which covers the posterior aspect of both bodies and discs, is the actual anterior boundary of the space; posteriorly the ligamentum flavum is spread over and between the vertebral laminae. On the lateral aspects of the extra-dural space the vertebral pedicles provide a discontinuous boundary which is punctuated by the intervertebral foramina (see Fig. 2.1).

The extra-dural space contains arteries, veins, lymphatics and fat, the relative and absolute numbers of which vary with age, cardivascular status, pregnancy and other factors. The spinal

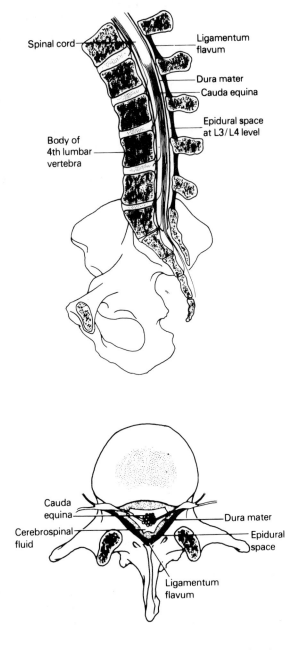

Fig. 2.1. Anatomy of the epidural space in the lumbo-sacral region.

nerves were not included in the list of contents because the dura is defined as the internal boundary of the extra-dural space, and a sleeve of dura and the other meninges accompany the nerve to at least as far laterally as the intervertebral foramen. This remains true caudally. Although the dural sac has its lower limit at about the level of S2, the remaining outflow of sacral nerves (the cauda equina) are individually ensheathed in dura, which eventually peters out as the filum terminale.

Many details of the anatomy of the extra-dural space, and of the structures with which it is intimately connected, have for long provided the basis of a controversy which is still not fully resolved. For a full and engagingly written exposition of this subject, the reader is referred to a recently published account (Bromage 1978).

Analgesia can be effected by the injection of local anaesthetic into the extra-dural space. In the light of the previous discussion, the implication is that the drug must penetrate the dura in order to reach the nerve fibres. The major site of penetration is the sleeve of dura which envelops the fully-formed spinal nerve. However, the presence in the cerebrospinal fluid of local anaesthetic or other substances injected into the extra-dural space, and the potential for passage of substances from within the subarachnoid space into the surrounding tissues, have been repeatedly demonstrated since the original studies of Brierley & Field (1948). Indeed, this report provided an important clue in the study of the natural history of poliomyelitis. There exists the potential that, to some extent, extra-durally administered analgesics act by virtue of their penetrance into the cerebrospinal fluid. The proportionate importance of this is, again, a matter of considerable debate, but few, if any, authorities claim it to be outstanding. Thus it is generally accepted that in order to achieve the desired effect, local anaesthetic given extra-durally must gain direct access to the appropriate spinal nerve as it approaches, or passes through, the intervertebral foramen.

This latter consideration presents the obstetric anaesthetist with the need, in theory at least, to make a two-pronged attack upon the extra-dural space As has been noted, the pain of the first-stage of labour is transmitted predominantly by impulses carried via nerves of root value T10-L1, whereas in addition sacral roots 2, 3 and 4 are involved in the pain of the second-stage. Several authorities, of whom Bonica (1967) is outstanding, advocated that this dilemma be met by adopting a two-pronged attack — the 'double catheter technique'. Others use a 'single prong' and rely upon a graduated flow of local anaesthetic solution to provide an appropriate sequence of nerve block, while yet others aim to achieve an extensive block throughout labour. The arguments for each technique will be developed later in this chapter.

Two routes of entry into the extra-dural space are available for obstetric analgesia: between two adjacent lumbar vertebral spines or via the sacrococcygeal membrane. The latter, which is termed the caudal approach, is now less-favoured. The technique of administering a caudal extra-dural block will be described, but thereafter more consideration will be given to the technique and outcome of the lumbar route.

Techniques of epidural analgesia

Caudal extra-dural block

Probably the most important step in the search for the sacral hiatus is to identify the mid-line, and this is best done by 'walking' down the tips of the spinous processes of the lower lumbar, and thence the sacral vertebrae. Eventually a gap will be appreciated, bounded laterally by the sacral cornua, which are the ends of non-fused posterior laminae of the lower sacral vertebrae. Caudal to this is the coccyx, which must also be identified. The beginner will find it useful to mark with a skin pencil the isosceles triangle which has as its base the line joining the sacral cornua and its apex the mid-point of the coccyx.

After appropriate preparation of the skin, local anaesthetic is infiltrated over the proposed site of entry into the cudal canal. This step is only necessary if it is intended to use a Tuohy needle for the purpose of introducing a cannula to provide a continuous caudal. For a single shot caudal, a disposable 20-gauge needle may be used and preliminary skin infiltration is not required.

The needle is inserted with its point directed slightly cephalad. It is advanced through the sacrococcygeal membrane — which offers a slight resistance — until it reaches the posterior aspect of the body of the underlying sacral vertebrae. The needle will have penetrated the periosteum. It should be withdrawn from the latter (a distance of 1 mm should suffice), and the shaft is then swung round so that the hub lies well within the natal cleft. There should be no resistance by tissues to this manoeuvre. The needle is then advanced up the sacral canal for a distance of 1—2 cm, again no resistance should be encountered. A 2 ml syringe is then attached to the needle and an attempt made to aspirate. If blood is obtained, the whole procedure should be repeated. If clear fluid is obtained, it must be assumed that the dural sac of the patient extends well below the level of S2, and has been pierced, and it would be wise to abandon the procedure.

If the aspiration test proves negative, the 2 ml syringe is filled with air and re-attached to the needle. Two fingers of the operator's left hand are placed lightly over the sacral hiatus and the air is injected through the needle. If no crepitus is felt, and the air is injected with minimal effort, local anaesthetic may then be administered or, alternatively, a disposable plastic catheter may be advanced through the Tuohy needle.

Under most clinical situations it is advisable that the patient be prone with the hips slightly flexed (a pillow under the pubic region helps) during initiation of a caudal but this is not very practical in the obstetric patient at term. For the pregnant patient the lateral position with the hips fully flexed is the preferred position. This makes identification of the surface markings more difficult, as the upper buttock distorts the line of the natal cleft.

Another practical difficulty associated with the procedure is the extreme variability of the bony anatomy of the sacrum. This has been extensively reviewed by Trotter (1947). The mean distance between the sacrococcygeal membrane and the posterior wall of the sacral vertebrae (the anterior-posterior diameter of the caudal canal) is 5.5 mm, but in five per cent of cases the distance is less than 2 mm, thus affording very little opportunity of threading a needle, particularly a Tuohy needle, up the canal after the initial entry has been gained. The density of the sacrococcygeal membrane is another variable; generally it is assumed to be virtually ossified in 5-8 per cent of subjects but this observation requires further evaluation. It was probably based upon examination of cadavers supplied to departments of anatomy, hence representing an elderly population. On the other hand, if the success rate claimed by practitioners of caudal analgesia in obstetric practice is a reliable guide, the incidence of failure to reach the caudal canal because of impenetrability of the sacrococcygeal membrane is much less than five per cent.

The danger of inadvertent dural puncture when performing a caudal has already been mentioned. Trotter (1947) reported that the distance from the upper limit of the sacral hiatus to the lowest extremity of the dural sac ranged from 16 mm to 75 mm, among subjects who did not have a spina bifida.

Another hazard associated with a caudal is that the needle might be advanced through the canal and through the sacrococcygeal joint during the initial manoeuvre. If this occurs, the rectum could be penetrated, a contingency which, of itself, is unlikely to cause much trouble. More seriously the fetal scalp or possibly skull might be penetrated if the fetal head has reached the perineum. This mishap has apparently occured on four occasions resulting in two fetal deaths (Finster et al 1965, Sinclair et al 1965).

The conduct of continuous caudal analgesia coincides so closely with that of continous lumbar extra-dural block that there would be little merit in detailing the two separately. By way of prologue, however, attention must be drawn to two important characteristics of caudal block. Firstly, it is inescapable that the sacral nerve roots will be blocked as a prelude to blocking the outflow which subserves uterine sensation. Secondly, in order for local anaesthetic to reach the T10–L1 spinal nerves a comparatively large volume of solution has to be injected. The capacity of the sacral canal alone may be as little as 12 ml or as much as 65 ml (Trotter 1947) but in practice, it is usually found that 20–25 ml of local anaesthetic solution will abolish the pain of labour. This may appear to be a surprisingly low volume in view of the range of values just quoted but probably reflects the fact that the sacral portion of the extra-dural space is partly taken up by venous distension as is the lumbar portion during pregnancy.

Lumbar epidural block

A. Techniques and complications of initiation

So far in this discussion the term 'extra-dural' has been used exclusively. Strictly speaking, the phrase 'lumbar extra-dural analgesia' should be employed. However, the term 'lumbar epidural' is now in common usage and will be the term used henceforth.

The usual approach to the lumbar epidural space is in the mid-line; a more lateral approach has been advocated (Carrie 1977) on the grounds that it avoids trauma to the supraspinous ligament while reducing the chance that the dura will be inadvertently punctured. There is certainly much to commend this paramedian approach, but it does not appear to have caught the active interest of most anaesthetists. The following detailed description of the technique will be confined to that which employs the mid-line.

A lumbar epidural can be initiated with the patient sitting, with back well bowed but in the pregnant patient, and certainly in one in labour, this is probably impractical as most anaesthetists take about 10–20 minutes from positioning the patient satisfactorily to insertion of an epidural cannula. However the sitting position for obese pregnant women is still advocated as it makes it less difficult to identify the bony landmarks of the mid-line.

The more usual position for pregnant mothers is the left lateral, but *meticulous attention to the precise positioning of the patient is of the most fundamental importance.* The lower half of the patient's back must follow the line of the edge of the bed or table and must be precisely vertical; her back must be flexed as much as is compatible with patient comfort. After the usual surgical cleansing of the selected site, infiltration of the skin, subcutaneous tissue and supraspinous ligament with local anaesthetic is undertaken. A preparatory entry is made through these structures with a sharp-pointed introducer, the point of entry being in the mid-line midway between two spinous processes which are reasonably well separated (usually the space between L2–L3, or L3–L4). The epidural needle is then advanced through this channel of entry in a slightly cephalad direction and absolutely parallel with the floor. The needle generally used is 16-gauge internal diameter, 18-gauge external diameter, which will allow a cannula to be threaded through. A Tuohy needle is the favourite choice, although a straight short-bevelled needle is successfully used by some anaesthetists.

The needle-point passes successively through skin then the supraspinous and interspinous ligaments to reach the ligamentum flavum. In many patients the supraspinous ligament is extremely tough, and as it has a smooth, rounded posterior aspect it tends to diver the needle from the desired direction. Considerable care must be taken to ensure that the direction does indeed remain true, by frequent lateral inspection of the shaft. The interspinous ligament offers little resistance, and entry into the more firm ligamentum flavum is usually easy to appreciate. This is the threshold of the epidural space, and from this point onwards anaesthetists will use a technique of their choice to identify the moment when the advancing needle-point enters the space.

There is a considerable number of techniques from which to choose, and a practitioner should gain a satisfactory familiarity with one and stick to it. They are all dependent upon the fact that the epidural space is a low pressure region. In the normal non-pregnant adult the pressure is slightly sub-atmospheric, in the pregnant woman it is somewhat higher (Messih 1981) but still offers very little resistance to the ingress of gas or fluid via the needle. The sequence of events is that a fall in resistance to pressure will be experienced during the advance of the needle as the point passes from the ligamentum flavum into the epidural space. A drop of fluid deposited within the hub of the needle or a column of fluid in a capillary tube attached to the needle will be 'sucked in' as entry into the epidural space is gained, or more accurately, the fluid is pushed in under the force of the atmospheric pressure which is usually sufficient in non-pregnant patients.

In the pregnant patient a higher positive pressure is required within the needle. The pressure is usually applied with the aid of a 10 ml syringe which contains air or fluid. Although fluid is used by many competent anaesthetists it is, in the writer's opinion, not the optimal choice for two reaons; it confuses identification of a possible dural puncture and it involves the possibility of injecting particulate matter, specifically powdered glass from the ampoule from which the fluid was obtained, into the epidural space. The use of air rather than fluid has neither of these hazards but the efficiency of this technique depends upon the syringe used. The plunger must be able to be moved smoothly through the barrel without much effort, the opposite of a syringe ideally used for aspirating blood, which requires a tight fit. Many anaesthetists insist that only a glass syringe is acceptable but there are makes of plastic disposable syringes which suit the requirements admirably. The pressure can be applied continuously or intermittently; with the latter technique pressure is applied afresh after each advance of the needle. Both are called the 'loss of resistance' technique.

The Macintosh balloon is used in another variant of this loss of resistance technique, when pressure is maintained continuously whilst the needle is being advanced. Although the equipment has not gained much popularity it is, in the writer's opinion, the finest discriminator of the precise moment of entry into the space. The soft-walled balloon is attached, by an intervening Luer-adaptor, to the hub of the needle when the ligamentum flavum has been reached. The balloon is inflated with air, and this provides a positive pressure of about 50 mmHg. When the needle-point enters the epidural space the balloon rapidly deflates.

When entry of the needle into the epidural space has been identified, a cannula is threaded through and the needle withdrawn. The length of cannula inserted through the needle should be such that 2–3 cm of it will have emerged beyond the needle-point; this can be assessed by reference to the identifying marks which are printed on most commercially available cannulae. Attempting to introduce a greater length of cannula into the space will only cause it to loop backwards and forwards as the tip meets resistance from veins and fat. For a similar reason it is doubtful that deliberate efforts to direct the cannula in either a cephalad or caudad direction are more successful than would occur by chance.

Local anaesthetic solution can be injected into the epidural space through the needle, either as a 'single-shot' technique or preparatory to inserting a cannula, a routine followed by many competent anaesthetists, but is not my practice for two reasons. First, a single-shot technique is not an appropriate choice for labour and, second, there is the possibility that the needle tip might be advanced through the dura whilst the injection is being made, producing a spinal block. Inserting a cannula does not add appreciably to the difficulties associated with initiation of an epidural and allows intermittent or continuous infusions of anaesthetic agents.

The final step is to attach a bacterial filter to the hub of the cannula. Although it has been argued that this device is not necessary (Abouleish et al 1977), it seems to be most unwise to risk the injection of solution contaminated with either bacteria or particulate matter into the epidural space, when the provision of this effective defence is so simple and relatively inexpensive (James et al 1976).

Three preliminary measures should be taken before the start of the procedure:

1. Determination of volume status. Assurance must be made that the patient is not hypovolaemic. This does not require the use of laboratory facilities, but merely a reasonable degree of clinical acumen. Thus a patient whose epidural is to be started in the morning, and who has therefore had little to eat or drink during the previous 12 hours, should be considered to be hypovolaemic, as should a patient who has been in strenuous labour for several hours without benefit of an intravenous infusion. Hypovolaemia is also a characteristic, some would say invariably, of pre-eclampsia though extravascular fluid may show as oedema. It is, therefore, essential to good practice that a patient with moderate or severe pre-eclampsia be given at least one litre of a crystalloid solution intravenously before the start of an epidural. Whether or not hypovolaemia is thought to be present, *it is an absolute rule that an* epidural is not to be started until an intravenous infusion is in progress.

2. Determination of blood pressure. Systemic blood pressure must be measured and recorded before the start of the procedure to provide a baseline recording and at regular intervals thereafter.

3. Determination of fetal heart rate. Monitoring of fetal heart-rate and uterine pressure must be in progress before and during initiation of the epidural. The time taken to complete the procedure may be 10–15 minutes but can be 30–40 minutes, the actual time in a given patient not being dependant upon the skill and experience of the anaesthetist but upon individual circumstance. It is important that monitoring be in progress throughout this time. If internal monitoring has not been established an external monitor must be applied.

Potential difficulties and complications. Those associated with inserting a catheter into the epidural space diminish with increasing experience of the administrator, but never disappear entirely. There would be little justification in discussing all the potential problems of epidural techniques in detail here; the performance of manual skills are best learned under supervision, during an 'apprenticeship', and not from books or journals. Three possibilities are, however, worthy of note:

1. Blood might appear in the needle or the cannula, and should be presumed to have come from a traumatised epidural vein. The incidence of this occurrence is probably of the order of 10 per cent. If blood continues inexorably to drip from the needle, or a considerable column advances up the cannula, entry into the lumen of a vein must be assumed and re-entry into the epidural space via an adjoining vertebral interspace undertaken. It is unusual for the complication to recur, but if it does it would be advisable to abandon the procedure.

2. Occasionally it proves to be difficult to thread the cannula beyond the length of the needle although confident entry of the needle-point into the epidural space has been gained. The likely explanation is that the space is narrow, and is possibly being encroached upon by a bulging dura. In this circumstance ask the patient to extend her hips very gently and slowly; if gentle pressure is applied to the cannula during this manoeuvre, there is a considerable chance that the cannula will suddenly begin to advance into the space as the tension on the dura relaxes. If this does not happen, there is no alternative but to withdraw the needle and try through an adjoining interspace.

3. The third complication is a dural tap. The incidence of this should be no more than two per cent in a well-organised service, but such an incident is virtually inescapable in even the most experienced hands. As noted already, the suggestion has been made that use of the paramedian approach reduces the likely occurrence of a dural tap (Carrie 1977). Husemeyer & White (1980) suggest that this is because there is a dorso-median fold of the dura which brings it in very close proximity to the ligamentum flavum precisely in the mid-line.

The dura can be punctured by either the needle or the cannula, although if the latter appears to have caused the breech it is possible that the dura was initially damaged by the needle. If clear, or slightly blood-stained, fluid is seen to drip from the needle or to travel up the cannula, it must be assumed to be cerebrospinal fluid (c.s.f.) unless proved otherwise. In most cases the anaesthetist will be fully aware that the dura has been punctured because of the 'feel' of the advancing needle. If there is doubt and it is thought that the fluid might be from a loculus of local anaesthetic, the fluid should be tested with paper strips sensitive to pH and glucose. If glucose is present in the fluid, the identification of c.s.f. has been made. However, the glucose concentration in the c.s.f. of a patient who has been fasting or undergoing considerable exertion can be low, so a negative test for glucose is not conclusive (Reisner 1976). In this situation the use of the pH paper aids the diagnosis; if the pH of the fluid is seven or more it should be considered to be c.s.f. but if five or less the fluid is likely to be local anaesthetic solution.

If an inadvertent dural tap is performed, the needle and/or cannula must be withdrawn and re-inserted via an adjoining vertebral interspace. It is most reprehensible to leave a patient with a dural tap yet without the benefit of epidural analgesia. *Local anaesthetic subsequently injected through a re-sited cannula will not enter the c.s.f. in any greater quantity than would have been the case had a puncture not been made.*

The complication of a dural tap is likely to be associated with headache. The incidence of 'spinal headache' is correlated with the size of the needle used, and, following an attempted epidural, is approximately 70 per cent (Crawford 1972). If no treatment is provided the headache typically will start on the day following delivery although it can become evident during labour; it is clearly postural in character, being virtually entirely relieved when the patient lies flat. Tinnitus ('popping in the ears'), nausea and vomiting are occasional accompaniments. In my experience of over

71

300 of these occurrences, following either a spinal anaesthetic or following an inadvertent tap, the headache, if left without active treatment, invariably persists for six days; this is succeeded by a day of 'muzziness' after which all symptoms disappear. Presumably this reflects the fact that it takes six days for the hole in the dura to heal. It is comforting to be able to assure a patient that her headache will clear spontaneously and permanently on a specified day.

In non-obstetric patients a 'spinal headache' frequently can be treated simply by bed-rest. Encouragement to take extra fluids is usually included in the management, but probably has very little merit. The great majority of post-natal patients cannot be treated in this way. There are two lines of active management currently practised:

1. An epidural drip is logically the first measure to be attempted. This consists of infusing a crystalloid solution (Hartmann's or Ringer's) into the epidural space via the filter and cannula. Institution of this infusion must be delayed until the requirement for epidural analgesia has passed, usually after the end of the third-stage of labour. The objective is the infusion of about 1.5 litres in 24–36 hours; despite the inclusion of the bacterial filter in the line this can be accomplished without undue difficulty. There is absolutely no requirement for the mother to be lying supine during this period. She can sit upright, feed her infant and take her meals, although it is probably better that she does not get out of bed. The infusion is stopped at a time convenient to the mother and the nursing staff, the cannula is withdrawn and tha patient may then resume her normal activities.

It is preferable that during the first 24 hour period after conclusion of the infusion the mother does not exert herself too energetically, and that she is given a laxative so that she does not require to strain at stool. In my experience the incidence of 'spinal headache', despite these measures, is approximately 35 per cent; the reason for success in the remainder is not easy to explain. Presumably equilibration of pressure across the dural perforation is sustained for long enough to permit the laying down of an initial sheet of protein upon which fibroblasts will subsequently weave the matrix of complete repair.

2. Epidural blood patching may be tried if the epidural infusion fails to prevent a 'spinal headache'. This measure was first described by Gromley (1960) and has gained considerable favour, the objective being to form a clot over the hole in the dura. After an epidural needle has been introduced into the lumbar epidural space, blood is withdrawn from the patient's vein and injected through the epidural needle. The needle is then withdrawn, a simple dressing is placed over the skin puncture, and the mother rapidly turns onto her back. She lies supine for 30 minutes to permit time for the blood clot to adhere to the dura, and then she sits. The headache will usually have gone.

Several features additional to this simple description are necessary to the safety and effectiveness of the measure. There must be no clinically apparent evidence that the patient has a bacteraemia, lest the infected blood leads to an epidural abscess. As a precautionary measure, sufficient blood should be withdrawn so that culture for aerobic and anaerobic organisms can be requested, thus providing an early warning of the presence of an infection which was not apparent at the time. The appropriate antibiotic sensitivity will also then be available. My own experience has taught me that a volume of up to 20 ml of blood should be injected in order to ensure that the hole in the dura is actually covered by the patch (Crawford 1980). The injection is made slowly and must be stopped immediately if the patient complains of a feeling of fullness in her back or of pain or discomfort in a leg — these symptoms are suggestive of distension within the epidural space and stretching of nerve roots.

The incidence of successful and permanent cure of 'spinal headache' by an epidural blood patch given in this way has been reported to be close to 100 per cent (Crawford 1980). It might be wondered therefore, why it is not used as the primary measure. The answer is that the technique of 'patching' is often used if the headache has complicated a single-shot *spinal* block. It, however, an epidural cannula has been in position, the drip as described above will fail to prevent a headache in only 35 per cent of cases; if a blood patch were first choice it would be employed unnecessarily in 65 per cent of cases. Although no serious complications of a blood patch have yet been reported, it is considered unacceptable that a large number be performed unnecessarily.

Injection of the blood directly through the cannula has been advocated, but has not proved to be very successful (Loeser et al 1978). Doubtless the reason for this is that, in many instances, the tip of the cannula (which will have been inserted via a different lumbar interspace from that through which the dural tap was made) is a considerable distance from the hole in the dura, and the injected blood does not cover it.

B. Test dose

It is customary to inject a test dose of local anaesthetic as a preliminary to establishing a block, the method varying between departments and individual anaesthetists. Probably the most commonly used technique is to inject 2 ml of 0.5 or 1.0 per cent lignocaine or a small dose of bupivacaine.

The objective of giving a test dose is to identify whether or not the cannula has been directed into an epidural vein or has transversed the dura. In the former circumstance the mother is likely to remark that her tongue tingles and that she feels a little light-headed; *such a report indicates that the cannula must be withdrawn and re-inserted.* There is less certainty that injecting a test dose is of use in identifying that the cannula is within the intrathecal space. Numbness and weakness of the legs might be experienced by the mother and thus provide the clue that the local anaesthetic has entered the c.s.f. but *the general consensus is that lignocaine in the concentration normally used is unlikely to produce a definitive response.* On the whole, anaesthetists are not greatly impressed by the practical results of using a test dose, but the routine is maintained partly as a matter of custom and partly because there appears to be no worthwhile alternative. One advantage of the procedure is that, by filling the cannula with local anaesthetic solution, it reduces the chance that the lumen will become blocked (by blood or by coagulated protein) before the first formal dose of bupivacaine or other drug of choice is injected.

C. Technique and complications of establishing a block

The following section must be preceded by a directive of outstanding importance. The ampoule containing the local anaesthetic which is intended to be injected as the first formal dose into the epidural space, or as a 'top-up' dose, must be checked by an independant witness. She must observe the contents of that ampoule being drawn into a syringe and observe the contents of that syringe injected through the sited epidural catheter and must countersign the appropriate prescription sheet to that effect. Only by such meticulous attention to detail will the disaster of administering the wrong solution be averted.

The local anaesthetic which is used in most parts of the world for lumbar epidural analgesia is bupivacaine. Chloroprocaine is favoured in North America because of its relatively brief latent period of onset, although its equally brief duration of action demands that either frequent re-injections are given or that bupivacaine is used subsequent to the initial dose of chloroprocaine. Chloroprocaine is not available for general clinical usage in the U.K. Following publication of reports of several cases of serious neurological damage, apparently consequent upon the inadvertent intrathecal injection of this drug (Corvino et al 1980), it seems unlikely that chloroprocaine will be released for general use in this country, although there is as yet no firm evidence that the drug itself was the cause of the neurotoxic effects.

Bupivacaine is commercially available in concentrations of 0.25 per cent and 0.5 per cent. Injection of the stronger solution is likely to provide not only more profound analgesia, but also a greater degree of motor-loss and depression of the 'bearing-down' reflex. By way of compromise, several anaesthetists mix the contents of the two concentrations to obtain 0.375 per cent solution, but this must be done by the anaesthetist and cannot be prescribed for 'midwife topping-up'.

Bupivacaine is obtainable as either a plain solution or in a solution containing adrenaline. The latter confers very little benefit to analgesia for labour, the adrenaline only prolonging the duration of activity of bupivacaine by about 10–20 minutes (Reynolds & Taylor 1971, Moir er al 1976); nor does it materially influence the maternal cardiovascular responses to injection into the epidural space (Broadfield et al 1975). The major deterrent to using bupivacaine plus adrenaline is that if, inadvertently, an injection is made into an epidural vein, the effect of the catecholamine could be catastrophic. Bearing in mind the previous tests to distinguish c.s.f. from drug solution it is noteworthy that the pH values of the plain solution is 6.1 whereas that of bupivacaine plus adrenaline is 3.0 (Bromage 1969).

If a patient is not in labour and the first dose of bupivacaine is intended to prevent pain at surgical induction, the mother should be reclining against a headrest during administration; this position should be maintained until the numbing effect of the local anaesthetic has been reported. On the other hand, if the mother is in labour when the epidural is started, she should be in the horizontal lateral position when the injection is made and 3–4 minutes later she should turn to her other side in order to attain bilateral distribution of the blocking effect. *Following the injection of local anaesthetic, the systemic blood pressure must be measured and recorded at 5 minute intervals for at least 15 minutes.*

There is likely to be a delay of 10–20 minutes before the mother begins to appreciate the effects of the first dose of bupivacaine but usually the extent of this delay is considerably reduced if the patient is in strong and painful labour at the start of the procedure. Subsequent doses (colloquially termed 'top-ups') will be effective much more rapidly, provided that the mother does not allow the analgesia to wear off to any marked extent.

Six undesirable responses can be encountered as a response to the first dose:

1. Hypotension. In clinical care this may be defined as a fall in systolic blood pressure greater than 20 mmHg. The step immediately to be taken if this occurs is to identify whether or not it is the result of the combined effects of vasomotor block and aorto-caval compression. Even if the mother was lying in the full lateral position when the fall of blood pressure was identified, she should be turned to the contralateral position, and this might effect a return to almost normotension. It is a useful gambit to ask the patient which side she has preferred to lie on during the final trimester. If she reports a marked preference for one side, the likelihood is that there will be less chance of her being hypotensive when she adopts that posture. If the blood pressure remains disquietingly low, despite a change of position, the intravenous infusion of Hartmann's solution should be speeded so that about a litre is given in about 20 minutes.

These measures will almost invariably succeed in remedying the situation. Rarely will any change in the pattern of the fetal heart-rate be observed as a result of the hypotension. If this does occur, the mother should be given oxygen to raise the transplacental gradient of partial pressure. If measures are taken to correct hypovolaemia before the epidural is started — and to prevent its occurrence subsequently — hypotension referable to vasomotor block should result from fewer than five per cent of all top-ups.

Administration of a vasopressor to correct the hypotension must be considered only if there is a dramatic fall of blood pressure with accompanying maternal and fetal distress; it should be regarded as a last resort. We have considered such drugs to be necessary for only eight of 25 000 labouring patients. *The vasopressor of outstanding choice in this circumstance is ephedrine.* Workers who have studied this subject extensively, have concluded that ephedrine is the vasopressor which, whilst being effective in reversing hypotension, is least likely to cause a reduction in utero-placental blood flow (Ralston et al 1974). The recommended dose is 5 mg i.v. although 10 mg might be required.

2. Injection of the local anaesthetic might produce absolutely no effect. Neither the anaesthetist nor the mother must be fooled into thinking that the patient is somehow 'resistant' to the action of the drug. Such dishonesty serves no useful purpose; the cannula must have been sited incorrectly. If time permits it should be re-inserted, for there is little point in fiddling around with the cannula in the hope of 'striking lucky'.

3. Unilateral block. This is a not infrequent response to the initial injection. Oftein it can be corrected by having the mother lie on the unblocked side and injecting another dose of bupivacaine. If the block continues to be unilateral despite this manoeuvre, the probability is that the cannula has been advanced too far anteriorly in the epidural space, and that there is a fibrous sheet or septum which interferes with the spread of local anaesthetic solution to the opposite lateral component of the space. Commonly it is possible to correct the error by withdrawing the cannula 2–3 cm. If this procedure is unsuccessful, the cannula must be inserted through an adjoining vertebral interspace.

4. The initial block is confined to one nerve root. This reflects the fact that the cannula has passed into or through a paravertebral foramen. Withdrawal of the cannula 2–3 cm will frequently correct the situation, but if it does not, the cannula must be re-sited.

5. Intravascular injection. Even when no blood is observed in the needle or cannula during insertion, it becomes evident, although infrequently, that the first dose of local anaesthetic has been injected directly into an epidural vein. More often than not, this occurrence will have become evident when the test dose is given. If this is not the case, the response to bupivacaine is likely to be rather more florid than that previously detailed with respect to lignocaine. As stated previously, although experience in the United States appears to be of cardiovascular collapse resulting from this mishap, in the U.K. the serious complication is usually a convulsion. Fetal distress due to the maternal convulsion and the placental passage of a bolus of drug is a likely accompaniment. There is sparse information about this event, as it is such a rare occurrence. If a convulsion does occur, or if the mother reports symptoms suggestive of a pre-ictal phase, the mother must promptly be helped into the horizontal lateral position and provided with supplementary oxygen via a face-mask. The episodes so far reported have been so brief that it appears to be unlikely that further active resuscitative measures would be required. However, the cannula must be removed and it would be prudent to abandon the attempt to provide an epidural for that mother. There is no evidence that an urgently conducted caesarean section would be of benefit to the fetus, which is likely to recover within a short time from any distress which it might have exhibited.

6. Intrathecal injection. The inadvertent intrathecal injection of a formal dose of bupivacaine is a rarity in a well-ordered department, but if it does occur it should occasion no great alarm and have no serious consequences. Characteristically, the onset of loss of sensation and of muscle power will be unexpectedly rapid, and the spread of the block is likely to be much more cephalad than anticipated. Only very rarely will there be accompanying respiratory embarrassment, and in my experience of such episodes the blood pressure remains surprisingly undisturbed. Therapy is required only if hypotension and respiratory embarrassment do become manifest; the former is treated as described previously, the latter by providing a continuous supply of oxygen to the mother. A severe degree of respiratory embarrassment will indicate the need to pass an endotracheal tube and assist maternal ventilation. This contingency is extremely remote, but the fact that it may exist provides the basis for the absolute requirement that *every practitioner who engages in epidural analgesia must be competent in endotracheal intubation, and must be satisfied that the instruments of intubation — plus immediately available oxygen — are present and in good condition in the area of operation.*

If an intrathecal injection is diagnosed, the cannula must be withdrawn and, at a suitable time, re-inserted so that an epidural block may be established after the effects of the spinal have worn off.

D. Maternal and fetal responses

A considerable amount of nonsense has been talked and written about the provision of lumbar epidural analgesia for labour. This stems mainly from a compulsion to treat the procedure as a science, which it is certainly not. Identical input does not produce identical results, and the range of variability of response is impressive. Whilst not a science, it is also not a matter relying upon mere chance. It is a craft. Like all crafts its successful application is based upon a few general guidelines and the accumulation of experience. After a suitably prolonged period of apprenticeship, an element of art begins to appear within the framework of the craft — that is, the more subtle tricks of the trade are learned and are employed when appropriate challenges are met.

Choice of dosage. The existence of these attributes are well exemplified by consideration of dosage. The volume and concentration of bupivacaine routinely injected at each top-up varies markedly between specialised centres. In some units 4–6 ml of 0.25 per cent bupivacaine is the routine dose, and the same volume of the 0.5 per cent concentration is substituted if analgesia has been insufficient. Reports from other units have referred to doses of 10–15 ml of 0.5 per cent or 15–20 ml of 0.25 per cent (Duthie et al 1968) and 7 ml of 0.5 per cent (Doughty 1969). Some practitioners, of whom the Brussels group are representative (Bleyaert et al 1979) almost invariably use a concentration of 0.125 per cent. In the author's hospital the standard dose is 10 ml, the first dose usually being of 0.5 per cent solution, and subsequent top-ups are generally made with 0.25 per cent.

The examples quoted are merely a small selection from those known to the writer. Each of the units referred to is staffed by informed and interested anaesthetists and obstetricians. Each group of specialists find the regimen followed in their respective units to provide very satisfactory results. The lesson to be learned is that there is no single 'correct dosage'. A corporate agreement is built up within the individual unit, which might have had its origin in the experience of an individual practitioner, or in sheer guesswork; the important point is that for them it works. If a satisfactory regimen has been evolved within a given unit, it is a mistake to try to 'graft-on' a markedly different regimen because it has proved to be successful elsewhere. The result of such an attempt is almost invariably disappointment (Stainthorpe et al 1978) and could conceivably prove to be disastrous.

Factors influencing spread. Local anaesthetic solution injected into the epidural space spreads by virtue of *volume displacement* and under the influence of *gravity*. In the main, the larger the volume injected the greater the spread, but this is not necessarily so; if the patient is sitting and the injection is made slowly, it frequently happens that gravity becomes the dominant factor.

Bromage (1962), in his classic report, identified the age and height of the subject as major determinants of the extent of segmental spread resulting from the injection of a standard dose. This was, however, a statistically-derived evaluation and in obstetric practice appears to have little relevance to clinical management, except possibly in reference to the care of either extremely tall or extremely short women. Pregnancy itself, as Bromage points out, is a factor of major influence. The pregnant woman requires approximately two-thirds of the volume of local anaesthetic which would be required by the same woman when she is not pregnant. The difference is undoubtedly related to the diminished available capacity of the epidural space due to venous distension. Aorto-caval compression will further reduce the available capacity. In like manner, the spread of a given volume of solution is potentially greater in the obese subject, reflective probably of excessive packing of the epidural space with fat (Hodgkinson & Hussain 1980).

Although it is the widely-held opinion that gravity is a major determinant of the direction of spread of injection solution, the view has recently been contested (Merry et al 1983). The proponents of this opinion suggested that capillary attraction is of greater importance in determining the direction of spread than is gravity. The question remains to be settled, but it is likely that, for the time being, most clinicians will, by encouraging appropriate posture of the mother, rely upon gravity as the determinant of direction of spread of block.

'Optimal spread'. The next point to be made in a general discussion of epidural analgesia is the extent of spread desired. Here there are two schools of thought. One is currently termed 'selective lumbar epidural block' (Hollmen et al 1977) or 'segmental block' (Gal et al 1979, Willdeck-Lund et al 1979). The objective is to attain a sensory block extending from T10 to T12, during the first-stage of labour, and to extend it to include the sacral roots only after the start of the second-stage. The advantages claimed for this technique are that, when comparisons are made with a more widespread block, there is a lower incidence of malpositions, required operative vaginal deliveries and maternal hypotension without a notable increase in failure to provide good pain relief (Jouppila et al 1979). The alternative is to permit — indeed, to encourage — establishment of a block extending from T10 to S5 as soon as possible after initiation of the epidural. The advantages claimed for this technique are that it markedly reduces the incidence of pain transmitted via the lumbar roots (specifically, of low back pain), and guards against the prospect that analgesia will be insufficient during the second-stage because of delay in achieving a satisfactory block of the sacral roots.

The contention that the latter technique is associated with a significantly greater incidence of maternal hypotension is difficult to sustain. The sympathetic outflow extends caudally only to the L2 segment, so the difference between the techniques is a matter of two autonomic nerve roots. Further, as has been already argued, hypotension due to vasomotor block alone should be a comparative rarity. Certainly, the provision of a widespread block from the beginning does evoke changes in the pattern of the delivery process, and these will be discussed in a succeeding section.

The relief from pain provided by an epidural is of high quality and impressive consistency. Almost every well-documented report from centres throughout the world refer to a success rate of 85–90 per cent. It is my experience — mirrored no doubt by others — that when bupivacaine 0.25 per cent is used, approximately half of the patients who have total analgesia will still be aware of their contractions, whilst the remainder will be completely oblivious of such sensations. In the former case, the awareness is that of distortion of the anterior abdominal wall by forward movement of the uterus during a contraction. When bupivacaine 0.5 per cent is used, the incidence of complete sensory loss is considerably higher.

Causes of failure

There is absolutely no justification for pretending to patients, other members of staff or the lay public that epidurals are invariably successful. In most well-organised units which conduct a large number of epidurals the incidence of failure to provide *any* pain relief lies between three and five per cent. Probably the major contributing factor to these failures is that the mother was too far advanced in labour when the epidural was attempted. When strong contractions are occurring every 2–4 minutes, the time taken to insert an epidrual cannula, whilst avoiding a dural tap, is comparatively long. Furthermore, as has been remarked, the first dose of bupivacaine will often take 10–20 minutes to become effective. Thus, in a considerable proportion of the cases in this category, the mother has been delivered before the epidural has begun to work and a 'failed epidural' must be documented. Understandably this is a source of displeasure not only to the patient, but also frustrates and annoys the anaesthetists (especially if it occurs in the early hours of the morning!). In my opinion an attempt should not be made to start an epidural for a mother whose labour has been progressing at a satisfactory rate and whose cervical dilatation has reached 9 cm if primigravid or 8 cm if multigravid. If, in these latter circumstances, regional analgesia is urgently requested, a spinal block should be given. Exceptions would be those patients whose partograph has 'levelled off' at 8–9 cm and who seem destined, if delivered vaginally, to have a rather difficult instrumental delivery. They are also probably becoming quite exhausted and an epidural is certainly indicated.

Two features most commonly associated with partial failure of an epidural are *missed segment* and *persistent backache*. A missed segment is a well-recognised complication which has not yet been satisfactorily explained. The incidence possibly varies slightly with the identity and concentration of the local anaesthetic used, but the condition occurs at least once in 6–7 per cent of labours, and in 1.5 per cent of labours it remains unrelieved throughout (Ducrow 1971, Bromage 1972). Most frequently it is unilateral but occasionally is bilateral. Typically, in my experience, it involves the first lumbar nerve root, and presents as pain in the area of the inguinal ligament coincidental with contractions. Injection of a higher concentration of the local anaesthetic, with the mother lying in the appropriate full lateral position, is frequently followed by elimination of pain. It is assumed that the nerve fibres involved have a perineural sheath which is more than usually resistant to diffusion of local anaesthetic.

Low backache, which tends to be continuous but becomes worse during contractions, is often associated with a 'flat sacrum' or a persistent occipito-posterior position. It is the most difficult of all the pains associated with labour to relieve by an epidural. It is transmitted by the lower lumbar and upper sacral roots. The mother should be in a reclining position when top-ups are given in an attempt to relieve the pain. More often than not the pain does not disappear until the fetal head has descended deeply into the pelvis.

Two other factors can give rise to pain during the course of an otherwise successful epidural: an *over-stretched bladder* and a *placental abruption*. The sensory supply of the urinary bladder has the root values S2, 3 and 4, and loss of bladder sensation is thus an unavoidable associate of an extensive epidural block. This need not, and indeed should not, lead to an increased incidence of catheterisation during labour. The advocate regimen is to ask the mother to empty her bladder voluntarily immediately before each alternate top-up, at a time when sensation is returning. Palpation suprapubically should however be routine to ensure that over-distension is not occurring. The discomfort or pain of excessive distension 'breaks through' an established epidural block, tends to be continuous and is felt in the suprapubic and perineal regions. This ability of the warning pain to pierce the block is a facet of the phenomenon referred to as the 'epidural sieve' (Crawford 1976).

Pain of pathological origin unassociated with normal uterine contractions can usually get through an otherwise well-established block. This aspect of an epidural is of importance during the labour of a patient with a uterine scar, as will be discussed later. It is also of relevance in an intra-partum abruption. If, in labour progressing under an effective epidural, the mother complains of persistent pain which is well localised within the surface marking of the uterus, the presence of a small abruption should be suspected. If this remains small, evidence of fetal distress is unlikely to occur and uterine activity will be unchanged, but subsequent examination of the placenta will usually reveal evidence of a retroplacental clot.

As a generalisation it may be stated that the effect of an epidural is insignificant upon uterine activity and the rate of progress to full cervical dilatation. If hypotension is avoided, and specifically if assurance is made that the mother is not exposed to aorto-caval compression, the introduction of bupivacaine into the epidural space will not lead to a change in frequency or strength of uterine contractions (Schellenberg 1977).

In clinical terms there is no significant difference in the duration of first-stage of induced or augmented labours between those conducted with, or without, an epidural. When labour has started spontaneously and is not stimulated, the first-stage will, on average, last one hour longer among 'epidural patients' than among 'non-epidural patients' (Studd et al 1980). These and other reported (Read et al 1983) statistical evaluations do not take into account the obverse: those cases in which the progress of labour is facilitated by an epidural. For patients in whom maternal exhaustion and distress are becoming prominent, an epidural will quite promptly lead to re-establishment of satisfactory progress (Maltau & Anderson 1975).

The fetal heart-rate pattern is equally unaffected by institution and maintenance of an epidural, provided again that maternal hypotension and/or aorto-caval compression are avoided. Occasionally, some diminution of beat-to-beat variability might be observed to follow a top-up, probably reflective of the placental transfer of bupivacaine, but this is of no significant import to the well-being of the fetus. Indeed the indirect effect upon the fetus can be beneficial. By ensuring freedom from pain and fatigue, maternal metabolic acidosis, and hence fetal infusion acidosis, is prevented.

However, it must be made clear that such advantage to the fetus is minimal in the great majority of cases. Considered in the context of normal clinical practice, in an estimated 85 per cent of labours the fetus is not notably compromised by either placental dysfunction or maternal exhaustion, and the provision of an epidural must not be advocated as being advantageous to the fetus in such circumstances.

A series of reports from Oulu, Finland, of studies of intervillous blood flow measured in human subjects using [133]xenon, have deepened considerably our understanding of the factors which can influence materno-fetal exchange of respiratory gases and metabolic products. A lumbar epidural administered to the normal parturient who is not exposed to aorto-caval compression and whose blood pressure is not significantly reduced, results in a slight but not statistically significant increase in intervillous and myometrial blood flow (Jouppila et al 1978, Husemeyer & Crawley 1979). Aorto-caval compression associated with the supine position will cause a significant decrease in intervillous blood flow whilst leaving myometrial blood flow only slightly diminished (Kauppila et al 1980). These relative changes are responsible for the fetal distress which so frequently becomes manifest when the mother is allowed to lie supine (Huovinen & Teramo 1979).

The effect of a lumbar epidural upon the intervillous blood flow of a patient with pre-eclampsia is much more dramatic and is described later.

The delivery process

The characteristics of the second-stage of labour and delivery are certainly altered by provision of an epidural. Contributing factors are the reduced tone of the pelvic floor muscle, the reduced power of the lower abdominal muscles and, though occurring less frequently, loss of the bearing-down reflex.

The *diminution of pelvic floor tone* reduces the facility with which the advancing fetal part rotates to the antero-posterior position, although this rotation can, in the majority of cases, eventually be accomplished spontaneously. *Reduction of muscle power in the lower abdomen* impedes the ability of the mother to bear down. The extent to which each of these two factors becomes operative is dependant to a significant degree upon the concentration of bupivacaine used for the top-ups late in labour. They will certainly be markedly apparent when the 0.5 per cent solution is administered, and can be insignificant if the 0.125 per cent solution is injected. In most labours a balance must be struck between a relative assurance of pain relief, which is afforded by the stronger solutions, and the avoidance of excessive loss of skeletal muscle tone and power.

The bearing-down reflex is obtunded because of a comprehensive block of the sensory side of the reflex arc. This occurs with rather more frequency when 0.5 per cent bupivacaine has been used than when the top-ups have been made with the 0.25 per cent solution, but the latter is still associated with an appreciable incidence of depression of the reflex. In my own experience, approximately 50 per cent of patients do not experience a bearing-down reflex. This does not mean that they are unable to bear-down, but certainly the expulsive effort is considerably diminished if reliance has to be place solely upon the voluntary components.

As a result of these features progress subsequent to full cervical dilatation is relatively slow. Contrary to earlier teaching, this does not of itself pose a hazard to fetal well-being.

Attenuation of this interval between full cervical dilatation and complete delivery has long been recognised as posing a hazard to both mother and infant. The danger to the mother was that of exhaustion, possibly compounded by postpartum haemorrhage due to uterine hypotonia, and infection. Neonatal asphyxia was the other component of the associated pathology. In their classic study, Pearson & Davies (1974) demonstrated an increasingly severe metabolic acidosis of both the mother and the fetus to be correlated with protraction of this period in cases in which the mother had retained the bearing-down reflex and, to a considerably lesser extent, in which the mother, being in receipt of an epidural, bore down only on request. The maternal metabolic acidosis undoubtedly reflects the fatigue and pain characteristic of a protracted delivery process, and is in turn responsible for the neonatal asphyxia and contributory to uterine hypotonia. Thus the impetus to deliver a mother who is poorly relieved of pain and who is becoming exhausted is both understandable and commendable. However, *when pain is not a feature and the mother does not have a reflex urge to bear down, there can be no justification for interference in the process of delivery unless there is compelling evidence of fetal distress or asphyxia.* The appreciable incidence of birth trauma as a result of mid-forceps, or low rotational forceps, delivery in the absence of fetal distress is a legitimate focus of criticism. There is no merit in encouraging the mother who has an epidural in progress to bear down voluntarily with contractions, at least until the presenting part is distending the perineum. The uterus of a mother who is not fatigued is an excellent propellant of the fetus, and the latter will accomplish its journey through the lower birth canal with deliberation, gently and safely if its progress is entrusted to the expulsive efforts of the uterus. (It is essential to note that throughout this period the mother must be safeguarded against aorto-caval compression, whether she be in the lithotomy position, the left lateral or reclining in a semi-sitting posture.) Understanding of this is increasing (Dorman & Wright 1983, Phillips & Thomas 1983, Read et al 1983, Maresh et al 1983) and should rapidly become more widespread. A simple lift-out forceps delivery might be deemed advisable once crowning of the fetal head has been achieved, but spontaneous delivery is a safely achievable objective in the care of a mother who is in receipt of a successful epidural (Bailey & Howard 1983). One further point is worthy of mention. Pressure of the advancing fetal part upon the pelvic floor causes an increase in the level of concentration of circulating oxytocin; this reflex can be blocked by an epidural given for labour and delivery (Goodfellow et al 1983). Therefore, if uterine activity appears to be flagging subsequent to full cervical dilatation, the judicious administration of a syntocinon infusion (or, if one is already in progress, an increase in its rate) is likely to be beneficial.

There are, of course, occasions when a low forceps or a mid-forceps delivery is required because of anatomical abnormalities or evidence of fetal asphyxia. In these circumstances the epidural proves to be beneficial because the relaxed pelvic floor and the absence of maternal pain enables delivery to be conducted with greater deliberation and gentleness than would otherwise have been the case.

Another maternal response, so far unmentioned, which is correlated to some extent with abolition of the bearing-down reflex is the feeling of 'deprivation'. The term is employed to describe the state of mind of the mother who reports that although she has been fully satisfied with the relief from pain provided by the epidural, she considers that she has missed part of the experience of labour and of full participation in the delivery. Analysis of unpublished data from the first 10 000 epidurals, given by myself and colleagues, showed that among primigravidae who retained the bearing-down urge, 1.3 per cent reported a feeling of deprivation, whereas 2.2 per cent of those who did not experience the reflex felt deprived. The respective incidences among multigravidae were 1.4 per cent and 2.9 per cent. It is, however, worth noting that of the mothers in this series who reported deprivation, 87 returned to the hospital for a subsequent pregnancy and only four of these declined the offer of a repeat epidural.

In what appears to be the only reported study of this response, Billewiez-Driemel & Milne (1976) found that among mothers interviewed 1 year after labour and delivery conducted under an epidural, 4 per cent concluded that they felt deprived.

'Pump epidural'

Because the required number of top-ups varies between three and six during a labour of average length, it was natural that consideration be given to the use of a continuous infusion of local anaesthetic into the epidural space. Logically, for this purpose, the local anaesthetic agent would be relatively short acting so that the effects of inadvertent overdose would rapidly wear off. It would also have low toxicity and a lower penetrance of the placenta. Procaine and chloroprocaine fulfil these criteria. However, the use of chloroprocaine in this manner has not been reported, and only one centre has reported on the use of procaine 2 per cent (Hunton 1979). The use of bupivacaine as 0.125 or 0.25 per cent solution has been described (Matouskova 1979, Taylor 1983). The results, while reasonably good, are by no means impressive.

The usual practice is to give a loading dose of the anaesthetic to initiate the block; thereafter the solution is given via a paediatric administration set or an infusion pump at a rate to maintain the required spread of analgesia. This can only be determined by trial and error. The tendency is for a larger total dose (in ml per hour) to be given than when the intermittent technique is employed, although the level of concentration of local anaesthetic in maternal and cord blood does not approach that associated with toxicity. The mother must be encouraged to turn laterally about every half-hour, and reasonably close monitoring of the blood pressure is necessary. Because bladder sensation is not appreciated it is necessary to ensure that over-distension is not allowed to occur.

On balance it appears that this technique is not labour-saving which was the primary objective of its introduction, and it affords few if any other advantages. Matouskova has summarised the technique as 'a practical, safe and simple method of obstetric analgesia', if the rules of its conduct are followed, but it offers no advantage over the method of intermittent topping-up.

Who should give the epidural?

Much sound and no little heat are generated during debates about whether or not obstetricians should be encouraged to give epidurals. The answers appear to be reasonably clear to the writer: in obstetric units which are served by enough competent anaesthetists there is little requirement or justification for the obstetricians to engage in the practice, except for purposes of training preparatory to going elsewhere. If there is a shortage of anaesthetists, who are able and willing to provide a service and to devote an appropriate amount of time to it, there can be no basis for criticising the practical involvement of obstetricians. But certain strict criteria must be fully satisfied. These are:

1. The obstetrician must have had the same extent of supervised experience in the technique and patient-management as an anaesthetist would have:

2. The obstetrician must be competent in, and prepared to undertake, cardio-pulmonary resuscitation in the unlikely, but nevertheless possible, event that his patient requires it. Thus the obstetrician must be capable of passing an endotracheal tube on a collapsed adult and experience of this manoeuvre should be gained under the tutelage of an anaesthetist. His personal standard of competence must be maintained by a brief 'refresher course' at 9–12 monthly intervals.

3. It must be understood and agreed by all the clinicians involved that if obstetricians do give epidurals to labouring patients this in no way allows the anaesthetic department to shelve its responsibility for providing an emergency service to the obstetric unit. There must be the continued assurance that informed and competent anaesthetic assistance will, without exception, arrive in the obstetric unit within, at the most, five minutes of the call for help. During that five minutes the initial supportive measures will have been undertaken by the obstetrician and the anaesthetist can then supervise or conduct any additional therapy which might be required.

There is no mystique attached to insertion of an epidural catheter and the maintenance of a continuous epidural for labour and delivery. Any obstetrician competent to perform a caesarean section or a vaginal breech delivery expeditiously will be little troubled learning the art and practice of epidural analgesia, but the aforementioned criteria must be met before he or she takes the reponsibility of a major service commitment in his own department. There are many excellent centres throughout the world in which these demands are fully met, including several in the U.K. (Taylor et al 1977, Ghosh-Ray 1980). Their existence should occasion no arguments about 'territorial rights', for in each instance the obstetricians concerned would gladly relinquish the epidural part of their practice if they were provided with an adequate service from the anaesthetic department.

Miscellaneous techniques

There are several techniques of pain relief which have proved to be relatively successful in other branches of medicine, such as the relief of chronic pain, and which have been applied with varying degress of success in obstetric practice.

Transcutaneous nerve stimulation. An electrical impulse is applied to the sensory nerves of the target organ using electrodes attached to the skin at appropriate sites. This has proved to be of some benefit during the first-stage of labour, although the incidence of complete relief from pain hardly exceeds the placebo effect. Relief during the second-stage has been of a poor quality (Robson 1979, Stewart 1979, Miller-Jones 1980) although it has been of help in relieving backache associated with labour (Bunsden et al 1981).

Acupuncture. The limited evidence available strongly suggests that this is ineffective in preventing the pain of labour (Wallis et al 1974).

Hypnosis. This can be extremely effective in eliminating the pain of labour, but in a small minority of patients. The claimed incidence of success ranges from 23–59 per cent among selected subjects (Moya & James 1960, Davidson 1962, Gross & Posner 1963). Other major drawbacks associated with this technique are the requirement to spend a considerable time with each patient during the ante-natal period and the heavy demands made by the hypnotised patient upon the midwifery staff of the delivery suite.

Abdominal decompression. This practice has had occasional advocates subsequent to its initial description by Heyns (1959). Its propensity to provide pain relief is said to be due to relaxation of the muscles of the anterior and posterior abdominal walls, whereby the uterus is able to move forwards freely during a contraction. Some claims for the effectiveness of the technique in providing analgesia (Leading Article Br. Med. J. 1968) have been disputed by others (Castellanos et al 1968). I would suggest the benefits are, in considerable measure, reflective of the mother's faith in the somewhat impressive apparatus. The claim that abdominal decompression is of appreciable benefit to fetal well-being has had considerable doubt cast upon it (Newman & Wood 1967).

Morphine and other narcotics. Although their use, when given extradurally for analgesia in labour, continues to excite interest, neither morphine nor pethidine has been reported to give very impressive results (Booker et al 1980, Skjoldebrand et al 1982, Writer et al 1981). Fentanyl offers the prospect of a better performance because it traverses the dura with greater ease. The duration of relief from the pain of uterine contractions has been reported as being longer after fentanyl (usually 80 μg) was injected epidurally than after bupivacaine (Justins et al 1982), but no longer than that following the i.m. administration of a similar dose of fentanyl (Justins et al 1983).

Although relief from contraction pain can be satisfactory, it has been found that extra-dural narcotics provide inadequate relief from the pain associated with delivery. Pruritis is a frequently reported complication of extra-durally administered narcotics. However, the most feared complication is delayed respiratory depression. The onset of this can be 8–12 hours after administration of the drug and its potential must inhibit application of this technique unless the mother is under constant informed surveillance throughout the critical period.

REFERENCES

Abboud T K, Sarkis F, Hung T T, Khoo S S, Varakian L, Henrikson E, Noueihead R, Gobelsmann U 1983 Effect of epidural anesthesia during labor on maternal plasma beta-endorphin levels. Anesthesiology 59: 1

Abouleish E, Amortegui A J, Taylor F H 1977 Are bacterial filters needed in continuous epidural analgesia for obstetrics? Anesthesiology 46: 351

Arthurs G J, Rosen M 1981 Acceptability of continuous nasal nitrous oxide during labour — a field trial in six maternity hospitals. Anaesthesia 36: 384

Bailey P W, Howard F A 1983 Epidural analgesia and forceps delivery: laying a bogy. Anaesthesia 38: 282

Baxi L V, Petrie R H, James L S 1979 Human fetal oxygenation following paracervical block. American Journal of Obstetrics and Gynecology 135: 1109

Beazley J M, Leaver E P, Morewood J H M, Bircumshaw 1967 Relief of pain in labour. Lancet 1: 1033

Belfrage P, Floberg J 1983 Obstetrical paracervical block with chloroprocaine or bupivacaine. Acta obstetrica et gynaecologica scandinavica 102: 245

Billewiez-Driemel A M, Milne M D 1976 Long-term assessment of extra-dural analgesia for the relief of pain in labour. II Sense of 'deprivation' after analgesia in labour: relevant or not? British Journal of Anaesthesia 48: 139

Bleyaert A, Sotens M, Vaes L, Van Steenberg A, Van der Donck A 1979 Bupivacaine 0.125 per cent in obstetric epidural analgesia. Anesthesiology, 51: 435

Bonica J J 1967 Principles & practice of obstetric analgesia and anesthesia Davies, Philadelphia

Brice J E H, Moreland T A, Walker C H M 1979 Effects of pethidine and its antagonists on the newborn. Archives of Diseases in Childhood 54: 356

Brierley J B, Field E J 1948 The connections of the spinal sub-arachnoid space with the lymphatic system. Journal of Anatomy 82: 153

Broadfield J B, Corall I M, Nicholson J R, Strunin L 1975 Cardiovascular changes in labour associated with extradural analgesia using bupivacaine. British Journal of Anaesthesia 47: 1291

Bromage P R 1962 Spread of analgesia solutions in the epidural space and their site of action: a statistical study. British Journal of Anaesthesia 34: 161

Bromage P R 1969 Evaluation of bupivacaine in epidural analgesia for obstetrics. Canadian Anaesthetists' Society Journal 16: 46

Bromage P R 1972 Unblocked segments in epidural analgesia for relief of pain in labour. British Journal of Anaesthesia 44: 676

Bromage P R 1978 Epidural analgesia, 2nd edn. Saunders, London

Bunsden P, Peterson L E, Selstam U 1981 Pain relief in labour by transcutaneous electrical nerve stimulation. Acta obstetrica et gynaecologica scandinavica 60: 459

Carrie L E S 1977 The paramedian approach to the epdirual space. Anaesthesia 32: 670

Caseby N 1974 Epidural analgesia for the surgical induction of labour. British Journal of Anaesthesia 46: 747

Castellanos R, Aguero O, De Soto E 1968 Abdominal decompression. American Journal of Obstetrics and Gynecology 100: 924

Cibils L A 1976 Response of human uterine arteries to local anaesthetics. American Journal of Obstetrics and Gynecology 126: 202

Cole P V, Crawford J S, Doughty A G, Epstein H G, Hill I D, Rollason W N, Tunstall M E 1970 Specifications & recommendations for nitrous oxide/oxygen apparatus to be used in obstetric analgesia. Anaesthesia 25: 317

Covino B G, Marx G F, Finster M and Zsigmond E K 1980 Prolonged sensory/motor deficits following inadvertent spinal anesthesia. Current Researches in Anesthesia & Analgesia 59: 399

Crawford J S 1972 The prevention of headache consequent upon dural puncture. British Journal of Anaesthesia 44: 588

Crawford J S 1976 The epidural sieve & MBC (minimum blocking concentration): an hypothesis. Anaesthesia 31: 1277

Crawford J S 1984 Principles & practice of obstetric anaesthesia, 5th edn. Blackwell, Oxford

Crawford J S 1980 Experiences with epidural blood patch, Anaesthesia 35: 513

Davidson J A 1962 Assessment of the value of hypnosis in pregnancy & labour. British Medical Journal 2: 951

Dolan P F, Rosen M 1975 Inhalation analgesia in labour: facemask or mouthpiece. Lancet 2: 1030

Dorman E M, Wright J T 1983 A prospective study on the second stage of labour following epidural analgesia. Journal of Obstetrics & Gynaecology 4: 40

Doughty A 1969 Selective epidural analgesia & the forceps rate. British Journal of Anaesthesia 41: 1058

Ducrow M 1971 The occurrence of unblocked segments during continuous lumbar epidural analgesia. British Journal of Anaesthesia 43: 1172

Duthie A M, Wyman J B, Lewis G A 1968 Bupivacaine in labour. Anaesthesia 23: 20

Evans J M, Rosen M, MacCarthy J, Hogg M I J 1976 Apparatus for patient-controlled administration of intravenous narcotics during labour. Lancet 1: 17

Evans J M, Hogg M I J, Rosen M 1976 Reversal of narcotic depression in the neonate by naloxone. British Medical Journal 2: 1098

Finster M, Poppers P J, Sinclair J C, Morishima H O and Daniel S S 1965 Accidental intoxication of the fetus with local anesthetic drug during caudal anesthesia. American Journal of Obstetrics and Gynecology 92: 922

Gal D, Choudry R, Ung K-A, Abadir A, Tancer M L 1979 Segmental epidural analgesia for labour & delivery. Acta obstetricia et gynecologica scandinavica 58: 429

Ghosh-Ray G, Taylor A B, Alberts F 1980 An integrated pain relief service for labour: co-operation between obstetricians, anaesthetists and midwives. Anesthesia 35: 510

Goodfellow C F, Hull M G R, Swaab D F, Dogterom J, Buijs R M 1983 Oxytocin deficiency at delivery with epidural analgesia. British Journal of Obstetrics & Gynaecology 90: 214

Gormley J B 1960 Treatment of post-spinal headache. Anesthesiology 21: 565

Greiss F C, Still J G, Anderson S G 1976 Effects of local anesthetic agents on the uterine vasculature & myometrium. American Journal of Obstetrics & Gynecology 124: 889

Gross H N, Posner N A 1963 Evaluation of hypnosis for obstetric delivery. Medical Journal of Australia 43: 819

Grundy E M, Zamora A M, Winnie A P 1978 Comparison of spread of epidural anesthesia in pregnant & non-pregnant women. Current Researches in Anesthesia & Analgesia 57: 544

Heyns O S 1959 Abdominal decompression in the first stage of labour. Journal of Obstetrics and Gynaecology of the British Empire 66: 220

Hodgkinson R, Hussain F J 1980 Obesity & the cephalad spread of analgesia following epidural administration of bupivacaine for Cesarean section. Current Researches in Anesthesia & Analgesia 59: 89

Hollmen A, Jouppila R, Pihlajiemi R, Karvonen P, Sjostedt E 1977 Selected lumbar epidural block in labour. A clinical analysis. Acta anaesthesiologica scandinavica 21: 174

Hughey M J, McElin T W, Young T 1978 Maternal & fetal outcome of Lamaze-prepared patients. Obstetrics & Gynecology 51: 643

Hunton J 1979 The use of procaine hydrochloride as a continuous lumbar epidural technique in labour. Anaesthesia 34: 274

Huovinen K, Teramo K 1979 Effect of maternal position on fetal heart-rate during extradural analgesia. British Journal of Anaesthesia 51: 767

Husemeyer R P, Crawley J C W 1979 Placental intervillous blood flow measured by inhaled ^{133}Xe clearance in relation to induction of epidural analgesia. British Journal of Obstetrics & Gynaecology 86: 426

Husemeyer R P, White D C 1980 Topography of the lumbar epidural space. Anaesthesia 35: 7

James F M, George R H, Naiem H, White G J 1976 Bacteriological aspects of epidural analgesia. Current Researches in Anesthesia & Analgesia 55: 187

Jones C M, Greiss F C 1982 Effect of labor on maternal and fetal circulating catecholamines. American Journal of Obstetrics & Gynecology 144: 149

Jouppila R, Jouppila P, Hollmen A, Kuikka J 1978 Effect of segmental epidural analgesia on placental blood flow during normal labour. British Journal of Anaesthesia 50: 563

Jouppila R, Jouppila P, Karinen J M, Hollmen A 1979 Segmental epidural analgesia in labour: related to the progress of labour, fetal malpositions and instrumental delivery. Acta obstetricia et gynecologica scandinavica 58: 135

Justins D M, Francis D, Houlton P G, Reynolds F 1982 A controlled trial of extradural fentanyl in labour. British Journal of Anaesthesia 54: 409

Justins D M, Knott C, Luthman J, Reynolds F 1983 Epidural versus intramusuclar fentanyl. Anaesthesia 38: 937

Kauppila A, Koskinen M, Puolakka J, Tuimala R, Kuikka J 1980 Decreased intervillous and unchanged myometrial blood flow in supine recumbency. Obstetrics & Gynecology 55: 203

Leading Article 1968 Abdominal decompression during pregnancy. British Medical Journal 2: 317

Loeser E A, Hill G E, Bennett G M, Sederberg J H 1978 Time vs success rate for epidural blood patch. Anesthesiology 49: 147

Maduska A L, Hajghassemali M 1978 Double-blind comparison of butorphanol & meperidine in labor. Canadian Anaesthetists' Society Journal 25: 398

Maltau J M, Anderson H T 1975 Epidural anaesthesia as an alternative to caesarean section in the treatment of prolonged exhaustive labour. Acta anaesthesiologica scandinavica 19: 349

Maltau J M, Eielsen O V, Stokke K T 1979 Effect of stress labour on the concentration of cortisol & estriol in maternal plasma. American Journal of Obstetrics & Gynecology 134: 681

Maresh M, Choong K H, Beard R W 1983 Delayed pushing with lumbar epidural analgesia in labour. British Journal of Obstetrics & Gynaecology 90: 623

Matouskova A 1979 Epidural analgesia: Continuous mini infusion of bupivacaine into the epidural space during labour. Acta obstetricia et gynecologica scandinavica suppl. 83

Meguiar R V, Wheeler A S 1978 Lumbar sympathetic block with bupivacaine: analgesia for labor. Current Researches in Anesthesia & Analgesia 57: 486

Melzak R, Taenzer P, Feldman P, Kinch R A 1981 Labour is still painful after prepared childbirth training. Canadian Medical Association Journal 125: 357

Merry A F, Cross J A, Mayadeo S V, Wild C J 1983 Posture and the spread of extradural analgesia in labour. British Journal of Anaesthesia 55: 303

Messih M 1981 Epidural space pressures in the lumbar region during pregnancy. Anaesthesia 36: 775

Miller-Jones C M H 1980 Transcutaneous nerve stimulation in labour. Anaesthesia 35: 372

Moir D D, Slater P J, Thorburn J, McLaren R, Moodie J 1976 Extradural analgesia in obstetrics: a controlled trial of carbonated lignocaine and bupivacaine hydrochloride with and without adrenaline. British Journal of Anaesthesia 48: 129

Morishima H O, Pederson H, Finster M 1978 Influence of maternal psychological stress on the fetus. American Journal of Obstetrics & Gynecology 131: 286

Moya F, James L S 1960 Medical hypnosis for obstetrics. Journal of the American Medical Association 174: 2026

Nelson M N, Enkin M W, Saigal S, Bennett K J, Milner R, Sackett D L 1980 Randomised clinical trial of the Leboyer approach to childbirth. New England Journal of Medicine 302: 655

Obstetric Analgesia and Anaesthesia

Nesheim B I 1983 Which local anaesthetic is best suited for paracervical block? Acta obstetricia et gynecologica scandinavica 62: 261

Newman J W, Wood E C 1967 Abdominal decompression & fetal blood gases. British Medical Journal 3: 368

Pearson J F, Davies P 1973 Effects of continuous lumbar epidural analgesia on the acid-base status of maternal arterial blood during the first-stage of labour. Journal of Obstetrics & Gynaecology of the British Commonwealth 80: 218

Pearson J F, Davies P 1974 Effect of continuous lumbar epidural analgesia upon fetal acid-base status during the first-stage of labour. Journal of Obstetrics & Gynaecology of the British Commonwealth 81: 971

Pearson J F, Davies P 1974 The effect of continuous lumbar epidural analgesia upon fetal acid-base status during the second-stage of labour. Journal of Obstetrics & Gynaecology of the British Commonwealth 81: 975

Phillips K C, Thomas T A 1983 Second stage of labour with and without extradural analgesia. Anaesthesia 38: 972

Ralston D H, Shnider S M, De Lorimer A A 1974 Effects of equipotent ephedrine metaraminal, mephentermine & methoxamine on uterine blood flow in the pregnant ewe. Anesthesiology 40: 354

Read M D, Hunt L P, Anderton J M, Lieberman B 1983 Epidural block and the progress and outcome of labour. Journal of Obstetrics & Gynaecology 4: 35

Refstad S O, Lindbaek E 1980 Ventilatory depression of the newborn of women receiving pethidine or pentazocine. British Journal of Anaesthesia 52: 265

Reisner L S 1976 Epidural test solution or spinal fluid? Anesthesiology 44: 451

Reynolds F, Taylor G 1971 Plasma concentrations of bupivacaine during continuous epidural analgesia in labour: the effect of adrenaline. British Journal of Anaesthesia 43: 436

Robson J E 1979 Transcutaneous nerve stimilation for pain relief in labour. Anaesthesia 34: 357

Schellenberg J C 1977 Uterine activity during epidural analgesia with bupivacaine. American Journal of Obstetrics & Gynecology 127: 26

Scott J S 1970 Obstetric analgesia. American Journal of Obstetrics & Gynecology 106: 959

Scott J R, Rose N B 1976 Effect of psychoprophylaxis (Lamaze preparation) on labor & delivery in primipara. New England Journal of Medicine, 294: 1205

Shnider S M, Abboud T K, Artal R, Henrikson E H, Stefani S J, Levinson G 1983 Maternal catecholamines decrease during labor after epidural anesthesia. American Journal of Obstetrics & Gynecology 147: 13

Sinclair J C, Fox H A, Lentz J F, Fuld C L, Murphy J 1965 Intoxication of the fetus by a local anesthetic. New England Journal of Medicine 273: 1173

Skjoldebrand A, Garle M, Gustafsson L L, Johansson H, Lunell N O, Rane A 1982 Extradural pethidine with and without adrenaline during labour: wide variation in effect. British Journal of Anaesthesia 54: 415

Stainthorpe S F, Bradshaw E G, Challen P D, Tobias M A 1978 0.125% bupivacaine for obstetric analgesia? Anaesthesia 33: 3

Stewart P 1979 Transcutaneous nerve stimulation as a method of analgesia in labour. Anaesthesia 34: 361

Studd J W W, Crawford J S, Duignan N M, Rowbotham C J F, Hughes A O 1980 Effect of lumbar epidural analgesia upon cervimetric progress & the outcome of spontaneous labour. British Journal of Obstetrics & Gynaecology 87: 1015

Taylor A B W, Abukhalil S H, El-Guindi M M, Watkins J A 1977 Lumbar epidural analgesia in labour: a 24-hour service provided by obstetricians. British Medical Journal 2: 370

Taylor H J C 1983 Clinical experience with continuous epidural infusion of bupivacaine at 6 ml per hour in obstetrics. Canadian Anaesthetists' Society Journal 30: 277

Trotter M 1947 Variations of the sacral canal: their significance in the administration of caudal analgesia. Current Researches in Analgesia & Anesthesia 26: 192

Tunstall M E 1961 Use of a fixed nitrous oxide & oxygen mixture from one cylinder. Lancet 2: 964

Wallis L, Shnider S M, Palahnuik R J, Spivey H T 1974 An evaluation of acupuncture analgesia in obstetrics. Anesthesiology 41: 506

Wiener P C, Hogg M I J, Rosen M 1977 Effects of naloxone on pethidine-induced neonatal depression. British Medical Journal 2: 228

Wiener P C, Hogg M I J, Rosen M 1979 Neonatal respiration, feeding & neurobehavioral state. Anaesthesia 34: 996

Willdeck-Lund G, Lindmark G, Nilsson B A 1970 Effect of segmental epidural block on the course of labour & the condition of the infant during the neonatal period. Acta anaesthesiologica scandinavica 23: 301

Writer W D R, James F M, Wheeler A S 1981 Double-blind comparison of morphine and bupivacaine for continuous epidural analgesia in labor. Anesthesiology 54: 215

3

Caesarean section

The principles which govern the choice of anaesthesia for caesarean section are identical with those referable to all obstetric practice: safety and comfort for the mother and avoidance of hazard to the child. However, under general anaesthesia the mother should be truly unconscious throughout the surgical procedure, and efforts to render and maintain her asleep must inevitably increase the prospect that the neonate will exhibit the effects of drug-induced depression. This is avoided if an epidural is used.

Anaesthetic techniques

There are four techniques of anaesthesia for caesarean section which are worthy of serious consideration; *general anaesthesia, lumbar epidural analgesia, spinal analgesia* and *local infiltration analgesia*. Of these, the last is likely to be employed when the general medical officer or obstetrician works without medical assistance, e.g., in undeveloped areas of the world.

Anaesthesia for caesarean section can best be considered with reference to elective section in a mother in good general and obstetric health and without evidence of placental dysfunction. This might be called the '*Group A elective section*' — patients who contribute to the series of mothers upon whom observations may be made to ascertain the relative merits of anaesthetic techniques without modification from other sources.

Certain measures should be employed in the case of these patients irrespective of the technique of anaesthesia:

1. Pre-operative medication

The prospect of undergoing an operation does not appeal to many people. Pre-operative apprehension can reasonably be expected in many of the mothers who are about to be delivered by elective caesarean section. There is little or no justification for not relieving this anxiety, however this must be accomplished without involving unacceptable depression of the infant. The oral administration of 5 mg diazepam one hour before the anticipated time of induction of anaesthesia satisfies these provisos (Crawford 1979).

Its prescribing should not be a routine measure, being a contradiction in terms for a mother who has opted to be awake during her section.

The prescribing of a tranquilliser does not relieve the anaesthetist of the obligation to visit the mother pre-operatively to reassure her. Such a visit is intended not only to enable the anaesthetist to ascertain that there are no untoward characteristics of the patient which might complicate the smooth running of the anaesthetic procedure, but also to give him the opportunity of describing in detail each of the steps in the pre-anaesthetic preparation of the mother. These visits are all too infrequently undertaken in the U.K.

2. The provision of blood

The volume of blood lost at caesarean section cannot be anticipated with precision, as it may vary from 300 ml to 3000 ml; the amount of loss is not closely correlated with the experience or expertise of the obstetric surgeon. Generally, there is a greater volume of blood loss if the placenta is low-lying or is situated anteriorly. In contrast to most surgical procedures, by far the greatest proportion of the total amount of blood lost throughout the operation is shed within a period of a very few minutes.

At least two units of cross-matched blood should be made available before the start of anaesthesia; if this is impossible, two units of Group O Rh negative blood must be obtained. The blood should be inspected, and its identification checked, by the anaesthetist before the start of anaesthesia, and it should not be returned to the blood-bank refrigerator until it has become evident, during the course of operation, that it will not be required. If there is reason to anticipate that blood loss will be considerable — as in the circumstances noted above — four units of blood should be made preparatorily available. Blood substitutes are not a satisfactory compromise.

This precautionary measure necessarily involves two other requirements: (a) an intravenous infusion of a crystalloid solution must be started *before* the induction of anaesthesia, (this applies whether general or regional techniques are employed); and (b) a satisfactory blood-warming device must be available in the operating suite as the blood will have been stored at 4°C.

3. Precautions referable to the gastrointestinal tract

It has been customary for many decades that food and drink should not be consumed by a patient during the six hours prior to the start of an elective surgical procedure. The basis upon which this rule was formulated is lost in the mists of antiquity. It probably derives from observation of patients who, presented for urgent operation, had suffered trauma or an episode of shock, had received a narcotic analgesic or had some gastrointestinal pathology. There is increasing evidence that, in obstetric departments at least, too many of our patients are put to unnecessary distress by being starved. There are grounds for valid criticism of the current practice whereby a mother is given a hospital meal at about 7 p.m. and nothing more up to the time that she is transported to undergo an operative procedure 14–16 hours later. Our practice now for mothers due to have an elective section is to offer them a light snack — tea, toast, biscuits, etc. — at 10.30–11.00 on the evening before operation. I personally encourage those who are to have a section under epidural, or are to have labour electively induced under epidural, to have a similar light refreshment at any time up to 7.30 a.m., as neither operative procedure is likely to be started before 10.30–11.00 a.m. It must also be borne in mind that the commonly adopted regimen results in the patient reaching the anaesthetic room in a somewhat dehydrated and possibly hypovolaemic condition. In consideration of this, it is becoming the practice to administer 500–1000 ml of a crystalloid solution intravenously in the anaesthetic room whilst the preparations for induction of general ·anaesthetic are proceeding. The situation is even more critical when regional analgesia is to be administered, as will be discussed later.

Pre-operative starvation increases, rather than diminishes, the likelihood that the gastric contents will be highly acidic. It is thus essential that an antacid be prescribed in order to guard against the hazard of the acid-aspiration syndrome. The much debated topic of antacid prophylaxis will be detailed in the next chapter. Reference is therefore limited to the statement that the writer's advocacy is that 15 ml of magnesium trisilicate mixture BPC should be given to the mother immediately before she is taken from the ante-natal ward, and a second similar dose administered just before the induction of anaesthesia, be it general or regional

4. Journey tilt

There is now general appreciation of the danger to both mother and fetus from aorto-caval compression. But it should also be appreciated that the fetus is likely to be at hazard even when adoption of the supine position by the mother does not result in maternal hypotension. It has been demonstrated that if the mother is transported from the ward to the anaesthetic room in the supine position, then tilted laterally until delivery of the infant, both mother and infant tend to be more acidotic than is the case if the mother is left in the lateral position from at least the time she leaves the ward (Crawford et al 1973). A possible explanation is that if she is supine during the journey, the reduced perfusion of the pelvis and legs encourages a local accumulation of metabolites which are released into the general circulation when a lateral tilt is subsequently provided. It is thus advisable that the mother lies on her own bed or trolley in the full lateral position throughout her journey to the operating suite.

The induction of general anaesthesia

When the patient is placed on the operating table in the anaesthetic room, care must be taken to ensure that the uterus is not compressing the aorta or the inferior vena cava and this may be accomplished in several ways. First, the operating table can be tilted laterally but this manoeuvre is unpopular because the mother might slip off the table. Secondly, the uterus can be displaced from the major vessels either manually or with the aid of a mechanical device (Colons-Morales 1970); this is a somewhat awkward technique which has found favour in North America but not in the United Kingdom. Thirdly, the mother's pelvis and abdomen may be tilted laterally by inserting a bolster or wedge under one side (Crawford et al 1972). Anatomical considerations suggest that the preferential direction of tilt or of uterine displacement should be to the patient's left, and it has indeed been demonstrated that aorto-caval compression occurs significantly more frequently when the patient is tilted to the right (Buley et al 1977). In practice however, it has been observed that under general anaesthesia, the choice of direction appears to be of little importance to the well-being of the infant. This is a generalisation, and no doubt there are occasions when the direction may be critical. If there is doubt about the matter, and if the condition of the fetus is already precarious, the mother should be asked if she has a preferred side to lie on when going to sleep during the final trimester; if she has, that is the appropriate direction to tilt her.

Avoidance of aorto-caval compression is essential if intra-uterine asphyxia is not to develop during the course of the operation, and failure to ensure this would be regarded as substandard practice. Protestations about the difficulties it might present to the operator are not acceptable reasons for failing to apply this precautionary measure.

Whilst the intravenous infusion of a crystalloid solution is being started, and the pre-operative blood pressure recorded, the mother should be encouraged to breathe from an oxygen source, via either a mask or mouth-piece, held by herself; the period of such pre-oxygenation should be at least 5 minutes. Its objective is primarily to safeguard both mother and infant against the period of apnoea which inevitably occurs between the onset of skeletal muscle paralysis and the start of artificial ventilation via an endotracheal tube.

Atropine (1.2 mg) or hyoscine (0.4 mg) is administered intravenously by many anaesthetists immediately before induction of anaesthesia. The anti-cholinergic drug is of benefit in preventing the salivation and bradycardia which may be evoked by suxamethonium.

Before the induction agent is injected, cricoid pressure should be applied. As a preliminary, the mother must be warned of what is about to happen, and told that it is a precautionary measure for the sake of her infant. Two fingers are placed on the cricoid cartilage, and pressure is applied in an antero-posterior direction. The objective is to block the lumen of the oesophagus and thus to guard against gastro-oesophageal regurgitation. The pressure must be firm but need not be so excessive that the mother believes she is being throttled. Applications of cricoid pressure can so distort the local anatomy as to render visualisation of the vocal cords difficult. To reduce this hazard it is advisable that counter-pressure be exerted on the back of the mother's neck by the assistant who is applying cricoid pressure, or that a block of firm foam rubber be placed under her neck as a preparatory measure. *Pressure must be maintained without remission from before the start of induction of anaesthesia until the endotracheal tube has been passed into the trachea and its cuff inflated.* This extremely important manoeuvre obviously cannot be conducted by the anaesthetist and assistance is essential. This is a critical period in the care of the mother and infant, and the provision of assistance to the anaesthetist takes precedence over every other activity in the operating suite. If the assistant is unsure how to apply cricoid pressure, the anaesthetist should give a clear, preparatory demonstration and might choose to delineate the surface markings of the cricoid cartilage on the mother with a crayon.

Endotracheal intubation is a highly advisable component of the technique. Another essential is a reliable and tested suction apparatus in the anaesthetic room.

Currently the the technique of anaesthesia is based upon a four-step procedure: (1) intravenous induction; (2) the use of suxamethonium to permit the rapid accomplishment of endotracheal intubation; (3) maintenance of skeletal muscle paralysis to allow controlled ventilation; (4) the maintenance of anaesthesia with volatile, and in some instances intravenous, agents.

Oxygen is administered in a relatively high concentration at least until the infant has been delivered. The somewhat limited evidence available (Rorke et al 1968, Marx & Matteo 1971, Robertson et al 1974) suggests that, for fetal well-being, the optimal concentration of oxygen to be administered to the mother is 67 per cent — less is likely to be insufficient, more will induce utero-placental vasoconstriction. This opinion has received support from a comparison of analyses of arterial blood obtained from anaesthetised pregnant women with those of similar samples from non-pregnant women subjected to the same technique of anaesthesia (Lyons & Tunstall 1979).

A detailed discussion of the relative merits and advocated dosage of induction agents including *thiopentone, methohexitone, etomidate, diazepam* and *althesin* will be found elsewhere (Crawford 1984). It is likely that thiopentone (250–300 mg) remains the most popularly used. Two agents should probably be avoided: *ketamine* because it causes a rise in blood pressure, and *methohexitone* because its short duration of action in the low doses required for obstetrics invite maternal awareness. A review of the skeletal muscle relaxants will be found in the same source, as will a discussion of the relative merits of the maintenance agents. Of the former group *alcuronium, atracurium* and *pancuronium* are better avoided because of the evidence suggesting placental transfer (Abouleish et al 1980, Ho et al 1981, Frank et al 1983).

It has been appreciated for many years that a small proportion of mothers delivered by caesarean section under general anaesthesia can recall some of the events of the operation, or give evidence of sub-clinical awareness by reference to 'unpleasant dreams'. The reported incidence has ranged from zero to 80 per cent but in recent years has rarely been reported to exceed 5 per cent (Crawford 1984). Probably only 10 per cent of the patients who have such recall will declare that pain was a feature of the episode and most will have recollections of only sound and touch. However, as Tunstall (1979) has demonstrated in a remarkable study, the fact that the mother does not recollect the events of her operation does not give assurance that she was unconscious throughout the procedure. It is apparent from Tunstall's report that the incidence of wakefulness is considerably greater than had been supposed. This poses the ethical problem of whether or not measures which might be potentially harmful should be taken to ensure that a patient is guarded against an unpleasant episode of which she will, in the majority of cases, have no subsequent recollection.

The dilemma is real and further compounded by the consideration that maternal distress caused by any wakefulness can induce fetal asphyxia (Morishima et al 1978). The choice therefore lies between the potential disadvantage of drug-induced neonatal depression and neonatal acidosis secondary to maternal distress. There can be no doubt that awareness during operation can be a horrifying experience, as testified by a harrowing personal account (Editorial 1979). Efforts to reduce the incidence by deepening the level of anaesthesia, by administering, for example intravenous agents is not the solution because most patients who have experienced awareness do so before delivery and such techniques would increase fetal depression. Not much success has attended attempts to induce retrograde amnesia by giving the mother a central depressant immediately after delivery (Barr et al 1977). Diazepam (5 mg orally) given as a pre-medication appears to be of some help in reducing the potential of awareness (Crawford 1980) but is unlikely to be invariably successful. The results of a recently completed extensive study have convinced us that the inclusion in the inspired mixture (70:30 oxygen : nitrous oxide) of either 0.5 vol per cent halothane or 0.3 per cent trichlorethylene reduces the incidence of maternal awareness virtually to zero, without demonstrable increase in the extent of intra-operative blood loss or noteworthy resultant neonatal depression (Crawford, Davies & Lewis, awaiting publication). If slight neonatal depression does result, it will be rapidly corrected when the infant excretes the volatile agent via its lungs.

When this technique of general anaesthesia is employed, the length of time which elapses between induction of anaesthesia and delivery of the infant (the I–D interval) plays a relatively minor role in determining the condition of the infant at delivery. The longer the interval, the more likely is it that there will be mild neonatal depression, as evidenced by a less than perfect Apgar-minus-colour score at one minute and an increased incidence of 'time to sustained respiration' (TSR) greater than one minute, but recovery will be rapid. There is thus no justification for reckless surgical speed in an effort to shorten the I–D interval in the absence of severe fetal distress. If fetal distress develops prior to surgical delivery the possibility of aorto-caval compression must be remembered and corrected, rather than indulge in surgical heroics. Failure to observe this complication will invoke the hazard of fetal asphyxia, the severity of which will increase with lengthening of the I–D interval and which is of much more serious import than drug-induced depression.

The time which elapses between the initial incision into the myometrium and complete delivery of the infant (the U–D interval) is more directly related to birth asphyxia. The longer the U–D interval, the greater is likely to be the severity of neonatal metabolic and respiratory acidosis (Crawford et al 1973, Downing et al 1976). As a generalisation it may be said that if the U–D interval is less than 90 seconds the infant will probably not have been rendered undesirably acidotic, but an extension of the interval beyond 90 seconds will place an increasingly heavy burden of asphyxia upon the neonate. The reason for this has now become apparent, as will be detailed later. It is most likely to be due to reflex vasospasm of the maternal vessels supplying the intervillous space, causing a reduced efficiency of exchange of respiratory gases between mother and fetus.

Epidural analgesia

Regional analgesia for caesarean section had a somewhat hesitant start because of the uncomfortably high incidence of maternal hypotension occurring when either epidural or spinal block was administered. There was also a discouraging incidence of failure in providing complete relief from pain and discomfort throughout the operation.

Complication of maternal hypotension

The introduction of two points of technique have greatly helped to avert the complication of hypotension: *pre-loading of the circulation* and the meticulous *avoidance of aorto-caval compression*. Pre-loading is necessary to permit the smooth accommodation of the circulating volume to the increased vasodilatation which inevitably results from an extensive vasomotor block. Without preloading, hypotension will occur and intervillous blood flow will diminish (Huovinen et al 1979). Plasma substitute is the agent successfully used by some clinicians (Huovinen et al 1979), but in my opinion is not advisable, because it is likely to remain in the circulation as the extensiveness of vasodilatation diminishes, thus reducing the efficiency of the auto-regulation of the circulating volume. The preferred method is to infuse 1–2 litres of crystalloid solution preparatory to initiation of the block. As the effects of the block begin to wear off and vasomotor tone returns, the rate of urinary output will increase considerably, hence maintaining a normal circulatory volume. Indeed it is important to remember and ensure that the bladder does not become over-distended.

Avoidance of aorto-caval compression is as important in preventing both maternal hypotension and perinatal acidosis as when general anaesthesia is used (Datta et al 1979), and the direction of tilt is more critical (James et al 1977). Again the logical choice of tilt is to the left but in about 10 per cent of patients this will be associated with a fall in blood pressue which will be corrected by tilting the mother to the right. The appropriate direction must be sought by the anaesthetist as the block is being initiated, but again a hint may be provided by enquiring of the patient which side she has, in recent weeks, preferred to lie on.

One other modification of technique has proved of benefit in further reducing the incidence of hypotension and of partial block failure: the procedure of incremental injections of bupivacaine (0.5 per cent) into the epidural space (Thorburn & Moir 1980, Crawford 1980). The first dose of bupivacaine (preferably 10 ml) is administered whilst the patient is sitting or semi-sitting; after about 10 minutes the mother lies horizontal in a lateral position and a further 10 ml bupivacaine is injected. Some 10 minutes later she turns onto her other side and a further dose of bupivacaine is injected, the amount being dependent upon how high the block has extended.

The advantage of this method is two-fold. Firstly, by inducing a gradual extension of the vasomotor block it allows time for a physiological adaptation of the maternal vascular system to proceed, and is less likely to produce hypotension than is the rapid onset of widespread vasodilatation induced by a single-shot technique. If this technique is used and aorto-caval compression avoided, the incidence of hypotension should be virtually zero. In the unusual circumstance that the maternal blood pressure does drop, ephedrine, 5 mg intravenously, is the vasopressor of choice. It is unlikely that a reduction in intervillous blood is associated with this technique, although such a reduction has been demonstrated to result from the use of the single-shot method (Jouppila et al 1978). Secondly, the technique of incremental dosage ensures that there will be an effective sensory block of the sacral and lower lumbar nerve roots, and thus avoids the discomfort, or pain, which previously was frequently complained of when the uterus was being sutured. There is an important point to be made here. In the interests of maternal and fetal safety the initiation of an epidural block for elective section will take a considerable length of time. Atempts to hasten the procedure by giving larger incremental doses, or by injecting more anaesthetic solution before the full extent of sensory block of the previous dose has been achieved, or, even worse, by injecting an assumed total dose requirement as a single shot, is an invitation to maternal hypotension, nausea and vomiting, with accompanying fetal acidosis. It is unlikely that, under normal circumstances, the mother will be ready for the start of surgery less than one hour after the start of the entire procedure.

The obstetrician must accept this and organise his clinical activities accordingly.

The total dose of bupivacaine required to provide an effective block appears to be of little consequence to the well-being of either mother or infant, though effective analgesia is unlikely if less than 25–30 ml bupivacaine (0.5 per cent) has been administered. In our hospital series we have administered in excess of 40 ml to a considerable number of mothers with no resulting maternal or perinatal complication.

A 5–6 l per minute flow of oxygen, directed into a lightweight mask loosely applied to the mother's face, from the time of the establishment of the block until delivery of the infant, is unlikely to be distressing to the mother and might be associated with a superior level of acid-base status of the infant at delivery although there is no firm evidence to support this hypothesis.

Mother's reactions post-delivery

Possibly the most undesirable feature for the mother who undergoes elective section under epidural analgesia is boredom and unease subsequent to delivery of the infant. Once the pleasure associated with delivery has subsided, there is a tendency for the mother to be concerned about relatively minor irritations such as immobility of her legs, some stiffness in the shoulders, or the length of time that the remainder of the operation is taking. It is, of course, the primary function of the anaesthetist to prevent or alleviate this emotional reaction, by intelligently directed light conversation and attention to the minor details of the patient's comfort. Light music from a cassette recorder may also be useful. It is, however, of even greater benefit to have the husband present throughout the operation. Not only does this add to the family enjoyment of the birth, but also the father's presence is invaluable in supporting the morale of the mother during the somewhat protracted final stages of the operation, which otherwise tend to be an anti-climax as far as the patient is concerned.

If the mother does become emotionally distressed, without evidence of experiencing pain from the operation, the slow intravenous injection of a dilute solution of diazepam, 5 mg, will frequently rectify the situation.

The duration of the U–D interval, which significantly affects the clinical condition and acid-base status of the infant when the section is conducted under general anaesthesia, has little apparent effect under an epidural (Crawford & Davies 1982). We postulate an explanation that the vaso-motor reflex referred to previously is prevented by the block of sympathetic and parasympathetic fibres induced by the epidural. There is also a possibility, yet to be examined, that under fairly light general anaesthesia manipulation of the uterus stimulates a surge of maternal catecholamine production which contributes to the constriction of vessels supplying the intervillous space. The lesson to be drawn from this contrast will be detailed later.

It is the experience in most centres that a proportion of mothers who have been given an apparently satisfactory epidural will complain of discomfort, sometimes of considerable pain, shortly after delivery. On occasion this is accompanied by nausea and vomiting. Often the discomfort is localised to the epigastrium, occasionally it is more extensive. It typically starts when the marsupialised uterus, or its visceral peritoneum, is being sutured. It is not invariably associated with rough handling of tissues, although that can be a contributory factor. Several measures have been employed in an attempt to alleviate the distress: a further epidural top-up with 1.0 per cent lignocaine, the administration of Entonox or pethidine, or, very infrequently, a general anaesthetic superimposed upon the epidural. As yet there appears to be no agreed successful policy. Swabbing the peritoneal cavity with 30 ml of a solution of 0.5 per cent lignocaine after the myometrial wound has been repaired has been proposed as a useful measure, but remains to be well tested. It would be a rational choice if the symptoms are due to vagal stimulation caused by traction on the peritoneum. If nausea is the sole symptom, the intravenous administration of 12.5 mg prochlorperazine (Stemetil) is usually an effective therapy. Nausea and vomiting are much more likely to occur if the mother is given an oxytocic and 'routine' ergometrine should not be used unless absolutely indicated. Such indications are likely to be present in fewer than one per cent of sections. The administration of ergometrine will undoubtedly provoke nausea and vomiting, and cause the mother's blood pressure to rise considerably, with an attendant headache, thereby negating the advantage of the entire procedure. If syntocinon is injected as a bolus, maternal nausea and vomiting will again be likely responses, but the blood pressure will fall. In the unlikely event that an oxytocic is required, infusion of a dilute solution of syntocinon should be given.

The choice between general anaesthesia and epidural analgesia

The choice is dependent upon several factors:

1. Maternal preference

A proportion of patients prefer to be unconscious during the section and, in the absence of any contraindication to general anaesthesia, this should be respected. On the other hand, a growing number of mothers are greatly attracted by the prospect of being able to see the infant at the moment of delivery, of being able to hold it and even put it to the breast after the cord has been clamped.

A comparative study of the levels of circulating beta endorphins demonstrated that mothers undergoing elective section under an epidural were less stressed than those who had been given a general anaesthetic (Abboud et al 1983).

2. The wish of the obstetrician

Many obstetricians in the United Kingdom may express uneasiness at the prospect of operating on an awake patient. This attitude is difficult to understand because, among all the practitioners of surgical skills, obstetricians are those who have most experience of caring for an awake patient under critical circumstances. Increasing experience of performing caesarean sections upon patients under an epidural usually serves to reduce, and eventually to eliminate, the disinclination of obstetricians in this matter.

3. Effect upon the fetus

For patients in whom there is no pre-operative evidence of placental dysfunction, the condition of the infant is likely to be only marginally better if delivered under epidural block than would be the case if the mother were given a general anaesthetic. The advantage attached to an epidural is more significant in patients with medical or obstetric problems causing fetal acidosis, because there is no risk of drug-induced neonatal depression being superimposed.

A further important factor relates to the U–D interval, where, as detailed above, prolongation beyond 90 seconds is associated with an increased incidence of clinical depression and asphyxia of the neonate if the section is performed under general anaesthesia, but appears not to be the case when an epidural is employed. In many cases there is no indication that the U–D interval will be prolonged. However, in the following categories it may take a considerable time after incising the uterus to deliver the infant: breech presentation, multiple pregnancy, scarred uterus (previous section or myomectomy), pre-term delivery (poorly-formed lower segment), very large infant. In each of these situations, concern for the infant's well-being dictates the choice of an epidural. It is of course in precisely these situations that some obstetricians feel most diffident about complying with the mother's request for an epidural, because of their concern that they will arouse maternal anxiety if the delivery proves to be difficult. The response to that is simple: the mother should be reassured that because there might be such difficulty it is better for the sake of her baby that she should have an epidural, and it will be the anaesthetist's role to sustain the mother's morale during the delivery process whilst the obstetrician devotes his entire attention to the procedure.

As previously remarked, the presumed or identified presence of placental dysfunction should mitigate in favour of an epidural. Pre-eclamptic toxaemia would fit well into this category, with two provisos; *if there is an associated coagulation defect an epidural should not be given, and if the mother is under the powerful influence of anti-convulsant therapy, maternal restlessness might well interfere too much with the safety of the surgical procedure.*

4. Maternal complications

Potential difficulties in the safe and effective provision of either technique must influence the choice. For example, the patient who has a respiratory infection whether acute or chronic, or in whom endotracheal intubation is anticipated to be difficult, should preferentially be given an epidural. On the other hand, the patient with a pathological condition of the lumbo-sacral vertebrae or receiving prophylactic anti-coagulants might be better served by a general anaesthetic.

It is frequently asserted that the presence of an anteriorly-lying placenta, or of a placenta praevia, is a contraindication to providing an epidural. This is a somewhat illogical view because there is no way of determining before any delivery or operation what the extent of blood loss will be; it can be well in excess of two litres irrespective of placental site. If a relatively large haemorrhage is anticipated, the appropriate amount of cross-matched blood should be available within the operating theatre, and two intravenous infusions should be initiated before the start of surgery.

5. Post-operative pain relief

A further advantage attached to the choice of an epidural is that the established access into the epidural space can be used for post-operative pain relief, thus enabling the mother to be fully alert throughout her post-operative period. The volume required to prevent pain from the operative site is likely to be greater than that necessary to establish the initial block, because the capacity of the epidural space increases as the abdominal mass is diminished. Bupivacaine is again the drug of choice. If administered in a concentration of 0.125 per cent there is unlikely to be loss of bladder sensation or weakness of the legs. However, it is more frequently the custom to use the 0.25 per cent concentration and, under that circumstance, care must be taken to ensure that the bladder does not become excessively distended.

A further complication which we have encountered in a very few mothers is blistering of the heels and an incipient superficial bedsore. These undoubtedly reflect prolonged recumbancy — allied with loss of sensation — on the operating table and in the recovery room, and must be rigorously guarded against by general nursing care.

Spinal analgesia

Theoretically, there should be no difference in effectiveness and safety between spinal analgesia and epidural analgesia for caesarean section. The extent of spread of nerve blockade including sensory, motor and vasomotor fibres, should be the same in each case. Indeed with regard to neonatal status spinal block should have preference because a much smaller mass of local anaesthetic is used in the course of this procedure than when an epidural is given; this, in turn, gives it an added advantage over general anaesthesia (Hodgkinson et al 1978).

However, spinal block suffers from similar disadvantages to those inherent in single-shot epidural block. The full extent of vasomotor block is achieved rapidly, providing no opportunity for physiological adaptation, and the incidence of associated hypotension is thus considerable (Corke et al 1982). Also, most anaesthetists find it less easy to achieve the desired spread of sensory block with a spinal than with an incremental epidural, so that unsatisfactory analgesia is more frequent. I believe that most obstetric anaesthetists in the United Kingdom would consider spinal block to be a poor third choice of anaesthesia for caesarean section.

Emergency caesarean section

The technique of general anaesthesia for emergency section does not require modification from that routinely used for patients requiring elective section.

The choice and technique of epidural block for emergency section may be modified depending upon the character and management of the preceding period of labour. If an effective epidural is already in progress, it is obviously easier to extend it to provide adequate analgesia for the operation than to initiate an epidural, but safety must take precedence over speed. If the established block extends, as is most likely, only to the T10 level, the cautious administration of top-ups to provide a sensory block to T4–6 can take about 40 minutes if maternal hypotension is to be avoided, and must be accompanied by additional pre-loading of the circulation. The final decision will depend not only upon the considerations noted above, such as maternal and obstetric preference, but also upon the urgency of the situation. *If the condition of the fetus or the mother is so parlous that minimal avoidable delay is essential, the choice must be general anaesthesia.*

If an epidural is not in progress and there is no great urgency to deliver the infant, initiation of a block can be undertaken in the manner described for elective section. Under this circumstance, *despite the assurance that haste is not imperative, there will be an understandable temptation to proceed with less deliberation that is advisable.* Such a tendency to cut corners could well be self-defeating because of the attendant danger of maternal hypotension further complicating whatever condition had prompted the decision to conduct an emergency section (Milne et al 1979).

The most important consideration relating to anaesthesia for emergency section is the *danger of regurgitation and aspiration,* which can occur when the operation is conducted under regional block, but the incidence is low and the attendant danger small. This complication is primarily associated with general anaesthesia, constituting one of the major arguments favouring epidural analgesia in preference to general anaesthesia for caesarean section. But whatever the cause this complication deserves the most careful attention and will be dealt with in detail in the next chapter.

REFERENCES

Abboud T K, Noueihed R, Khoo S, Hoffman D I, Varakian L, Henrikse E, Goebelsman U 1983 Effect of induction of general and regional anesthesia for Caesarean section on maternal beta endorphin levels. American Journal of Obstetrics & Gynecology 146: 927

Abouleish E, Wingard L B, De La Vega S, Uy N 1980 Pancuronium in caesarean section and its placental transfer. British Journal of Anaesthesia 52: 531

Barr A M, Moxon A, Woollam C H M, Fryer M E 1977 Effect of diazepam and lorazepam on awareness during anaesthesia for caesarean section. Anaesthesia 32: 873

Buley R J R, Downing J W, Brock-Utne J G, Cuerden C 1977 Right versus left lateral tilt for caesarean section. British Journal of Anaesthesia 49: 1009

Colon-Morales M A 1970 Self-supporting device for continuous left uterine displacement during caesarean section. Current Researches in Anesthesia & Analgesia 49: 223

Corke B C, Datta S, Ostheimer G W, Weiss J B, Alper M H 1982 Spinal anesthesia for Cesarean section. Anesthesiology 37: 658

Crawford J S 1984 Principles & practice of obstetric anaesthesia, 5th edn. Blackwell, Oxford

Crawford J S 1979 Premedication of elective caesarean section. Anaesthesia 34: 892

Crawford J S 1980 Experiences with lumbar extradural analgesia for caesarean section. British Journal of Anaesthesia 52: 821

Crawford J S, Burton M, Davies P 1972 Time and lateral tilt at caesarean section. British Journal of Anaesthesia 44: 477

Crawford J S, Burton M, Davies P 1973 Anaesthesia for section: further refinements of a technique. British Journal of Anaesthesia 45: 726

Crawford J S, Davies P 1982 Status of neonates delivered by elective Caesarean section. British Journal of Anaesthesia 54: 1015

Crawford J S, James F M, Davies P, Crawley M 1976 A further study of general anaesthesia for caesarean section. British Journal of Anaesthesia 48: 661

Datta S, Alper M H, Ostheimer G W, Brown W U, Weiss J B 1979 Effects of maternal position on epidural anesthesia for cesarean section, acid-base status, & bupivacaine concentrations at delivery. Anesthesiology 50: 205

Downing J W, Mahomedy M C, Coleman A J, Mahomedy Y H and Jean D E 1974 Anaesthetic induction for caesarean section: Althesin versus thiopentone. Anaesthesia 29: 689

Downing J W, Mahomedy M C, Jeal D E, Allen P J 1976 Anaesthesia for caesarean section with ketamine. Anaesthesia 31: 883

Editorial 1979 On being aware. British Journal of Anaesthesia 51: 711

Frank M, Flynn P J, Hughes R 1983 Atracurium in obstetric anaesthesia. British Journal of Anaesthesia 55: 113S

Ho P C, Stephens I D, Triggs E J 1981 Caesarean section and placental transfer of alcuronium. Anaesthesia & Intensive Care 9: 113

Hodgkinson R, Bhatt M, Kim S S, Grewal G, Marx G F 1978 Neonatal neurobehavioural tests following cesarean section under general & spinal anesthesia. American Journal of Obstetrics & Gynecology 132: 670

Huovinen K, Lehtovirta P, Forss M, Kivalo I, and Teramo K 1979 Changes in placental intervillous blood flow, measured by the [133]xenon method during lumbar epidural block for caesarean section. Acta anaesthesiologica scandinavica 23: 529

James F M, Crawford J S, Hopkinson R, Davies P, Naiem H 1977 Comparison of general anesthesia & lumbar epidural analgesia for elective cesarean section. Current Researches in Anesthesia & Analgesia 56: 228

Jouppila R, Jouppila R, Kuikka J, Hollmen A 1978 Placental blood flow during caesarean section under lumbar epidural block. British Journal of Anaesthesia 50: 275

Lyons G, Tunstall M E 1979 Maternal blood gas tensions, physiological shunt & $V_D V_T$ during anaesthesia for caesarean section. British Journal of Anaesthesia 51: 1059

Marx G F, Matteo C V 1971 Effects of different oxygen concentrations during general anaesthesia for elective caesarean section. Canadian Anaesthetists' Society Journal 18: 587

Milne M K, Dalrymple D G, Allison R and Lawson J I M 1979 Extension of lumbar epidural analgesia for caesarean section. Anaesthesia 34: 992

Morishima H O, Pedersen H, Finster M 1978 Influence of maternal psychological stress on the fetus. American Journal of Obstetrics & Gynecology 131: 286

Robertson A, Fothergill R J, Hall R A, Bond R W 1974 Effects of anaesthesia with a high oxygen concentration on the acid-base status of babies delivered at elective caesarean section. South African Medical Journal 48: 2309

Rorke M J, Davey D A, Du Toit H J 1968 Fetal oxygenation during caesarean section. Anaesthesia 23: 585

Thorburn J, Moir D D 1980 Epidural analgesia for elective caesarean section. Anaesthesia 35: 3

Tunstall M E 1979 The reduction of amnesic wakefulness during caesarean section. Anaesthesia 34: 316

4

Regurgitation and aspiration: causes and management

Successive publications of the triennially-issued Reports of Confidential Enquiries into Maternal Deaths in England and Wales bear sombre testimony to the fact that, over the past two to three decades, anaesthesia has been increasingly identified as a major contributor to the deaths associated with an avoidable factor. This is related in part to the still-common problem of deploying inexperienced junior anaesthetic staff to obstetric units. This is not the full explanation however, as is evidenced by the experience of one London teaching hospital where during the period 1958–78 general anaesthesia was the commonest single cause of maternal death (Morgan 1980).

The most common feature associated with 'anaesthetic deaths' has been a mishap during induction of anaesthesia. Such mishaps predominantly include difficult or failed intubation, and vomiting or regurgitation with aspiration.

Failure to intubate successfully

It should be within the compass of any anaesthetist entrusted with an obstetric commitment to respond effectively and safely to this challenge. There is no shame attached to being unable to pass an endotracheal tube upon a particular patient; every anaesthetist will encounter several such subjects in the course of his professional career. The true test lies in knowing what to do and in being alert enough to do it quickly.

Every obstetric department in which anaesthesia is administered should have an agreed protocol, with which all medical, nursing and ancillary personnel in the delivery suite/operating theatre complex should be conversant, for dealing with this emergency. The protocols in general use are based upon the 'failed intubation drill' initially described by Tunstall (1976). The protocol in effect in the Birmingham Maternity Hospital is detailed in the accompanying table (4.1). A measure of its necessity may be

Table 4.1   Failed intubation drill

I   **Maintain cricoid pressure throughout**

II   **Do not persist**
Do not increase danger to mother and fetus by stubborn prolongation of attempt to intubate

III   **Call for help**
A   IMMEDIATE: theatre personnel, surgeons, etc
B   ANAESTHETIC: if available

IV   **Turn the patient fully on to her side** — PREFERABLY LEFT
Do **not** put head down: this splints the diaphragm and makes ventilation harder to carry out

V   **Maintain ventilation**
With oxygen via a face-mask
Using an oropharyngeal (or nasopharyngeal) airway if necessary
until the effects of suxamethonium have worn off

and USE A SUCKER IN THE MOUTH to aspirate any material which presents

IF OXYGENATION IS STILL IMPOSSIBLE:
CRYCOTHYROID PUNCTURE with 14-gauge Jelco catheter and entrain oxygen — see DIFFICULT INTUBATION KIT

ONLY IF DESPERATE: TRACHEOSTOMY

VI   **Anaesthesia**
IF SOME DELAY IS ACCEPTABLE use REGIONAL TECHNIQUE
1. Allow patient to awaken
2. Carry out **EPIDURAL (not** spinal)

or IF DELAY IS UNACCEPTABLE — SPONTANEOUS VENTILATION
1. Leave patient on her side
2. Maintain cricoid pressure throughout procedure
3. Maintain GA with spontaneous ventilation of a volatile agent
4. Keep patient on her side during surgery with SLIGHT head-down tilt
5. Use NASO-PHARYNGEAL airway if necessary

   RECOVERY
   a. Pass NASO-GASTRIC TUBE before recovery of laryngeal reflex
   b. Recover on her side

or IF BOTH ALTERNATIVES ABOVE ARE IMPRACTICAL

LOCAL INFILTRATION
1. With Lignocaine — done by surgeon
2. With patient awake and
3. Breathing oxygen throughout

gauged from the fact that in that unit which conducts 5000–5500 deliveries annually, including 500–600 caesarean sections (half of them emergencies) under general anaesthesia, a failed intubation at the hands of an experienced anaesthetist is encountered on average twice a year, and a difficult intubation, for which the help of a more experienced colleague is obtained, about four times a year.

The attention of obstetricians must be brought particularly to three features of the protocol:

1. This is an acute life-threatening emergency and delay of seconds can literally spell the difference between life and death. If the anaesthetist calls for help, it must be provided instantaneously, whether or not the obstetrician and assisting nursing staff are scrubbed and gowned. The manpower required rapidly to turn a pregnant women into the full lateral position whilst the anaesthetist is attempting to maintain her airway, and his assistant is continuing to apply cricoid pressure, is transparently obvious.

2. If anaesthesia can be maintained using a face-mask, whilst the mother breathes spontaneously (step VI), she must remain in the full lateral position and the obstetrician must conduct the section under such a circumstance without cavil.

3. There will be occasions when anaesthesia cannot be safely or successfully maintained and it is impracticable to provide an epidural, yet a section must be accomplished. A spinal block is unacceptable in this situation. Being a single-shot technique it might not extend high enough, which would compound the dilemma, or might extend so high that severe hypotension and respiratory embarrassment result — an invidious situation following upon a failed intubation. The course of action must be for the obstetrician to conduct the section under local infiltration.

The technique of local infiltration analgesia is relatively simple. Basically it consists of infiltrating with local anaesthetic solution each layer of tissue in the line of the next intended incision. It has been described in more sophisticated detail by Ranney & Stanage (1975), as follows.

The drug advocated was 1.0 per cent procaine without adrenaline; the total volume injected never exceeds 100 ml and is usually approximately 60 ml. As an alternative 1.0 per cent lignocaine could be used, but then the total volume must not exceed 60 ml. Possibly some clinicians would accept the use of 1.0 per cent lignocaine with adrenaline, which would permit the employment of a larger volume. Four skin weals are raised in the vertical line, 4 cm lateral to the umbilicus, extending from the level of the umbilicus

116

down to the pubis. Through this the local anaesthetic is infiltrated subcutaneously and beneath the fascia of the recti muscles to provide a rectangular field block. Four additional weals are raised along the line extending from the umbilicus to the symphysis pubis, from which subcutaneous infiltration of procaine is carried out. Following incision of the skin and fat in the mid-line, the rectus fascia is infiltrated, and after this has been incised the transversalis and peritoneum are infiltrated. A further 5–10 ml of local anaesthetic is injected beneath the peritoneum covering the lower uterine segment, and this is massaged around the myometrium of that region.

The mother is undoubtedly likely to feel some discomfort during the entire operative procedure, but that is a small price to pay for the life of herself and her baby. The technique was in common use among obstetricians three to four decades ago, before the availability of reasonably safe general anaesthesia became widespread. *It must be relearned by the new generation of obstetricians, because it is a life-saving measure.* Just as no trainee anaesthetist can be deemed worthy of undertaking full responsibility for the care of patients without being able to cope promptly and correctly with a failed intubation, so no trainee obstetrician can be deemed worthy of achieving similar status without demonstrating the capacity to perform, expeditiously and successfully, local infiltration analgesia for caesarean section.

It is possible that many of the deaths associated with difficulty at intubation were the result of a combination of hypoxaemia and reduced cardiac output, the latter being due to caval compression. Under non-obstetric circumstances, failure to intubate a previously healthy adult of child-bearing age is, in the absence of regurgitation/aspiration, a rare cause of death. Its relatively frequent fatal outcome in pregnant patients must therefore reflect an obstetric factor; the fact that the patients were lying supine during induction of anaesthesia and the associated syndrome of caval compression makes this the probably 'lethal' element.

Prevention and management of regurgitation and aspiration during induction of anaesthesia

Dietary management

The aspiration of gastro-oesophageal contents continues to cause the greatest concern in obstetric anaesthesia. The most common cause of maternal death used to be asphyxia due to obstruction of the upper respiratory tract by semi-solid or solid material. Appreciation of this problem led to the introduction of an advised dietary regimen during labour (Crawford 1956), based upon the knowledge that gastrointestinal function was depressed during active labour. The more protracted the labour the greater was gastrointestinal depression likely. Indeed, a review of case histories of maternal deaths previous to the mid 1950s reveals that in most of those associated with the aspiration of gastric contents the mother had been in prolonged labour. The advocacy therefore was, and is, a low fat, low residue diet. This was to be permitted to patients who had been in active labour for a short time and who, in view of their obstetric and medical history, were unlikely to require a general anaesthetic during their delivery. For patients who did not fulfil these criteria, and especially for those who had entered the phase of 'prolonged labour', oral intake was limited to sips of water. The clinical context in which this regimen was devised and practiced may be better appreciated by noting that the term 'prolonged labour' was defined as established labour continuing for longer than 18 hours in a primigravid patient and for longer than 8 hours in a multigravid; these periods were not infrequently exceeded in many obstetric units.

During the past decade there has been a marked tendency, apparently nationwide, to deny food and drink to all labouring women. In part this has been prompted by the general introduction of the 'active management of labour', which resulted in the mean duration of labour being reduced from 12–14 hours to 6–8 hours. However, despite the assumption of medical and nursing staff, a considerable proportion of labouring mothers do experience hunger. This is especially the case among those who have labour induced, or go spontaneously into labour in the morning following and overnight fast. The symptom becomes even more pronounced among mothers who are experiencing a completely pain-free labour, as one conducted under an epidural. There is no justification in denying a light diet to such mothers if they request it, or indeed in failing to offer refreshment to them, provided that there is no compelling contra-indication.

Labour of itself does not reduce the rate of gastric emptying. The important factors which do exert an inhibitory effect are: maternal exhaustion (which might be relieved by sustenance additional to intravenous fluids), unremitting pain and narcotic analgesics

(Holdsworth 1978). Under each of these circumstances oral intake is best restricted to sips of water. If clinical judgement indicates that there is a good chance that the mother will require general anaesthesia for delivery by caesarean section, a similar restriction should apply. Categories of such cases would include moderate or severe pre-eclampsia, fetal compromise identified pre-labour, and the premature breech (whether singleton or multiple). In most other circumstances there will probably have been 2–3 hours of advance warning that an emergency section may be required and that interval will allow sufficient time for the gastric contents to be passed into the small intestine.

The light diet referred to is designed for rapid assimilation and transport out of the stomach. This process is not hastened by the administration of metaclopramide in labour (Howard & Sharp 1973). There will, however, be situations in which the mother who requires urgently to be anaesthetised has recently taken a substantial meal, or has been in labour for an excessive length of time and is thus likely to have retained a considerable volume of material in her stomach. The anaesthetist will then consider the advisability of conducting gastric emptying. If such a measure is likely to prove life-threatening to either mother or child, for example, if there is active haemorrhage, or acute fetal distress, or a prolapsed cord, it will not be undertaken and a 'calculated risk' will be carried out.

Gastric emptying techniques

There are two procedures currently available for carrying out gastric emptying. One is effective and relatively unpleasant, the other is less effective and more distressing. *The inefficient alternative is the passage of a large gastro-oesophageal tube.* A considerable quantity of gastric contents may be siphoned up through the tube (provided that the bore is large enough and the contents sufficiently fluid), but some will be vomited as a reflex response to pharyngeal stimulation.

The advocated technique is to stimulate the vomiting centre with apomorphine. The procedure is simple. Apomorphine is dispensed in ampoules containing 3 mg of the drug in solution (it is no longer freely available commercially, but can be dispensed by the local pharmacy department, or, in case of difficulty may be obtained from the Department of Pharmacy of Huddersfield Royal Infirmary). The solution is drawn into a syringe and diluted to 10 ml with Hartmann's solution or any innocuous diluent. The mother sits on the operating table with a vomit bowl on her lap and is told what is about to happen. Apomorphine is slowly injected intravenously, and the injection is stopped as soon as the mother says that she feels sick — this usually happens when approximately 1 mg (3–4 ml) has been given. The patient will then vomit for about a minute. Immediately after the episode of vomiting, nausea will recur and the mother will salivate copiously. At this time atropine (1.0 mg) or hyoscine (0.4 mg) should be injected intravenously and the nausea and salivation will stop. An anti-cholinergic drug should not be given before the administration of apomorphine, as this causes prolongation of the periods of nausea before and after vomiting.

Well-conducted investigations (Holdsworth 1978) have confirmed the writer's personal observations that the apomorphine technique is much less distressing to the mother than is gastric intubation. Criticism of the technique is by no means muted, but appears to be poorly informed. It is probably based upon lack of conversance with the method, or the inappropriate use of apomorphine, such as the injection of an undiluted bolus. There is no evidence that the amount of administered dose which undoubtedly crosses the placenta is in any respect harmful to the fetus.

Once gastric emptying has been effected and a dose of antacid has been administered (a point discussed later), induction of anaesthesia may proceed in the manner previously described. *The provision of a ready source of suction and the correct application of cricoid pressure are mandatory.*

If obstetrician and anaesthetist agree that a calculated risk must be taken, and general anaesthesia induced without prior emptying of suspected stomach contents, a gastro-oesophageal tube should be passed after delivery of the infant, the contents siphoned off, antacid instilled into the stomach and the tube removed.

A rather curiously intense interest has been taken in the status of the gastro-oesophageal sphincter. The pressure gradient between stomach and oesophagus is diminished slightly in the majority of pregnant patients during the final trimester, but in a minority there is a considerable reduction of the gradient. The physiological gastro-oesophageal sphincter becomes grossly ineffective, the 'barrier pressure' is much reduced, and a situation similar to a hiatus hernia obtains; these are the patients who complain of 'heartburn of pregnancy'. It has been demonstrated that both atropine and hyoscine further reduce the barrier pressure (Brock-Utne et al 1977, Dow et al 1978), that metaclopramide increases it (Brock-Utne et al 1978), and that the fasciculations of the abdominal wall, induced in non-pregnant patients by suxamethonium, can increase the pressure gradient from stomach to oesophagus (Smith et al 1978). In the present writer's opinion, these observations, whilst interesting in themselves, are irrelevant to clinical practice. The obstruction — or lack of it — offered at the lower end of the oesophagus to the passage of material from the stomach cannot be considered consequential to the safety of the mother during induction of anaesthesia. Reliance must be placed entirely upon the effectiveness with which the lumen of the oesophagus is obliterated by the application of cricoid pressure.

The acid-aspiration syndrome

This remains the most formidable problem of all. It may be defined as a chemical bronchopneumonia resulting from the entry of acidic material into the lower respiratory tract. *It is the dominant form of morbidity and the major contributor to mortality among pregnant patients to whom a general anaesthetic is administered, although it is possible that, in recent years, difficult or failed intubation has been the major provocative factor.* It is often referred to by the name of the obstetrician who first described the syndrome (Mendelson 1946).

Considerable investigation has determined that the pH and volume of the aspirated material are important. The syndrome is very unlikely to result if the pH of the aspirated material exceeds 3.0 (Bannister & Sattilero 1962, Vandam 1965, Taylor & Prys-Davies 1966). If the pH value of the material is very low (e.g., 1.5-2.0) the entry of less than 20 ml could be sufficient to initiate a fatal response whereas several hundred millilitres of fluid of pH 3.0-3.5 initiates a benign course (Taylor 1975). *Appropriate prophylaxis requires that both the volume and acidity of the gastric contents be considered.* The former has already been discussed, and attention will now be paid to measures used to reduce intragastric acidity.

Antacid prophylaxis

As the acidity of the gastric contents is derived almost entirely from hydrochloric acid secreted from the gastric mucosa, a logical approach is to block this secretory mechanism.

The H_2 receptor blockers, cimetidine and ranitidine, have been intensively investigated in this regard. They undoubtedly have the property of reducing or inhibiting the production of gastric acid, but the timing of their administration is critical. When cimetidine (400 mg) is taken orally it must have been administered 90–150 minutes before the induction of anaesthesia in order to ensure that the pH of gastric contents will be above the critical level (Johnson et al 1983); when the intravenous route is chosen (200–300 mg) the time factor becomes even more constrained, perhaps 45–60 minutes (McCaughey et al 1981). Ranitidine has a longer duration of action than does cimetidine, but again the timing of dosage is all important to success; of 30 mothers given 150 mg by mouth on the evening before operation and another 150 mg orally 1–2 hours pre-operatively, none had gastric contents of pH lower than 2.5 at the start of the operation (Andrews et al 1982). Furthermore, neither of these drugs will neutralise acid present within the stomach. It seems likely that the role these agents have in averting the danger of acid aspiration is in the care of mothers who are to undergo elective section, and not in the care of labouring women (Johnson et al 1983).

The performance attributed to glyopyrrolate has proved to be even less impressive, even when this anticholinergic agent is given in combination with atropine (Dewan et al 1982).

Sodium citrate administered as a 0.3 molar solution in doses of 15–30 ml has proved to be considerably more reliable in the context of routine clinical practice. Its administration 10–47 minutes before elective section was associated with a safe level of intragastric pH in one study (Gibbs et al 1982). Its administration as a pre-anaesthetic 'top-up' to labouring women who have been treated with an H_2-receptor blocker has been advocated (Johnson et al 1983). Compared with magnesium trisilicate mixture, it acts as neutralising agent rather more rapidly, but its duration of effective activity is considerably briefer — 30–60 minutes as against 2 hours.

Colloidal aluminium hydroxide (Aludrox), a mixture of magnesium trisilicate and aluminium hydroxide (Gelusil) and a mixture of aluminium hydroxide and magnesium hydroxide (Mylanta II), have proved to be relatively ineffective unless administered in very considerable quantity. The antacid in most common use in delivery room practice in the U.K. remains magnesium trisilicate mixture BPC:

Magnesium trisilicate	500 mg
Light magnesium carbonate	500 mg
Sodium bicarbonate	500 mg
Peppermint emulsion concentrate	0.25 mg
Chloroform water, double strength	5 ml
Water to	10 ml

The advocated dosage of this mixture is 15 ml every 2 hours. There are two stipulations: (i) at least two doses must have been administered before the start of an anaesthetic to give greater assurance that any acid which had been accumulated in the stomach before the antacid regimen was started would be neutralised; (ii) a final dose must be given within 10–15 minutes of the induction of anaesthesia, irrespective of the timing of the last routine dose. Our study previously referred to (Crawford & Potter 1984) has made it clear that the mixture must be dispensed within the 4-week period following its preparation. Thus, reliance upon commercial preparations is, currently at least, not acceptable.

It must be appreciated that strict adherence to this regimen does not afford an absolute guarantee that the pH of the intragastric contents will be above the critical level at the time of induction of anaesthesia. As Holdsworth et al (1980) have demonstrated, layering of gastric contents could lead to the situation in which an appreciable quantity of acidic gastric contents is not permeated by the antacid. Interestingly, however, layering has also been observed in respect to mothers treated with cimetidine (Johnson et al 1983). On the other hand, such a consideration must not encourage a nihilistic approach. Failure to make reasonable assurance that the gastric contents are rendered alkaline, by the rigorous enforcement of an acceptable regimen of prophylaxis, must be construed as culpable negligence. The fact that each year in England and Wales alone, 7–10 mothers die of what is confidently diagnosed as the acid-aspiration syndrome, leaves no room for inattention to details, much less for complacency (D.H.S.S. 1979).

Recently, the opinion has been broadcast that antacid prophylaxis as at present practised, is of doubtful value because the aspiration of gastric material which includes the antacid, will itself cause severe and potentially fatal lung pathology. Experiments have been described in which the hydroxides of aluminium and magnesium instilled into the pulmonary tree of dogs resulted in severe damage to lung parenchyma from which recovery, if it occurred, was greatly protracted (Gibbs et al 1979); the responses were similar to those which followed the instillation of hydrochloric acid. In comparison, the instillation of saline and of sodium hydroxide caused relatively little damage. Studies such as these have prompted the view that the particulate matter contained in mixtures of commonly-used antacids is potentially as dangerous as gastric acid (Wheatley et al 1979). This opinion has received some support from clinical experience of aspiration of a mixture of magnesium hydroxide and aluminium hydroxide (Bond et al 1979), and from several somewhat poorly-informed comments on maternal deaths which have occurred in the U.K. On the other hand, accounts have been published of patients who have evidenced no pulmonary complication following aspiration of gastric contents buffered with antacid (Bassell & Gotha 1979). Possibly the most persuasive evidence was obtained from a survey of obstetric anaesthesia services in the Birmingham Region (12 per cent of the U.K. population) during a six month period (Crawford & Opit 1976). Aspiration of gastric contents was reported to have occurred in 22 cases (representing 0.90 per cent of the total general anaesthetics surveyed). The outcome is shown in Table 4.2.

Table 4.2 Outcome in 22 patients who aspirated gastric contents

| | | | Asymptomatic | |
	Died	Difficult resuscitation	No therapy	With therapy
No antacid or only one dose (9)	2	1	4	2
2 or more doses of antacid (13)	0	1 (2 doses)	8 (one with 2 doses)	4 (one with 2 doses)

No single preventative measure can be relied upon with certainty to guard a patient against the acid-aspiration syndrome. All the components aimed at prevention must be rigorously invoked; diet, antacid prophylaxis, gastric emptying if appropriate, immediately available suction, cricoid pressure, endotracheal intubation and informed assistance. There is increasingly persuasive evidence accumulating to suggest that the choice of regional analgesia in preference to general anaesthesia for caesarean section is the measure most likely to result in the elimination of maternal deaths from acid-aspiration. However, it requires to be emphasised that the choice of regional analgesia does not give absolute assurance that the mother is completely protected from the danger of

124

regurgitation/aspiration. Several maternal deaths due to this complication have been reported as having occurred whilst the patients were undergoing caesarean section under spinal analgesia (Klein et al 1953, Stearns & Frederickson 1957).

A full discussion of the treatment of a mother who has developed the acid-aspiration syndrome is beyond the remit of this book. However, the following points may be made here. If there is any suspicion that aspiration of regurgitated material has occurred, the reaction of a sample of the regurgitated material should be tested with pH paper (an item which should be a standard component of the furnishings of the anaesthetic trolley). If the pH is greater than 3.5 no remedial action is required unless the mass aspirated is causing respiratory obstruction. If the pH value is less than 3.5, the potential that the acid-aspiration syndrome will develop must be assumed. Ventilation of the mother with a mixture containing a high concentration of oxygen must be maintained. Bronchial lavage, or attempted neutralisation of the aspirated material are potentially hazardous procedures and strongly contra-indicated. If bronchospasm becomes evident, it must be relieved with an appropriate bronchodilator. Although the advisability of administering corticosteroids is doubted by some, most clinicians continue to advocate their use: either methyl prednisolone hemisuccinate (0.5–1.0 mg) or hydrocortisone sodium hemisuccinate (200–300 mg) i.v. immediately, followed by hydrocortisone 100 mg i.v. 6-hourly for 48 hours and 50 mg 6-hourly for a further 48 hours. Rapid completion of the operation followed by prompt transport of the mother to a properly equipped and staffed intensive care unit must be the rule: the mortality from this condition is probably of the order of 20 per cent.

REFERENCES

Andrews A D, Brocke-Utne J G, Downing J W 1982 Protection against pulmonary acid aspiration with ranitidine Anaesthesia 37: 22

Bannister E K, Sattilero A L 1962 Vomiting & aspiration during anesthesia. Anesthesiology 23: 251

Baraka A, Saab M, Salem M R, Winnie A P 1977 Control of gastric acidity by glycopyrrolate premedication in the parturient. Current Researches in Anesthesia & Analgesia 65: 642

Bassell G M, Gotha M N 1980 Pulmonary aspiration following antacid therapy (correspondence). Anesthesiology 52: 450

Bond V K, Stoelting R K, Gupta C D 1979 Pulmonary aspiration syndrome after inhalation of gastric fluid containing antacids. Anesthesiology 51: 452

Obstetric Analgesia and Anaesthesia

Brock-Utne J G. Dow T G B, Welman S, Dimopoulos G E, Moshal M G 1978 Effect of metaclopramide on the lower oesophageal sphincter in late pregnancy. Anaesthesia & Intensive Care 6: 26

Brock-Utne J G, Rubin J, McAravery R, Dow T G B, Welman S, Dimopoulos G E, Moshal M G 1977 Effect of hyoscine & atropine on the lower oesophageal sphincter. Anaesthesia & Intensive Care 5: 223

Coombs D W, Hooper D, Colton T 1979 Acid-aspiration prophylaxis by use of preoperative oral administration of cimetidine. Anesthesiology 51: 352

Crawford J S 1956 Some aspects of obstetric anaesthesia. British Journal of Anaesthesia 28: 201

Crawford J S, Opit L J 1976 A survey of the anaesthetic services to obstetrics in the Birmingham Region. Anaesthesia 31 Supplement & summary (p 56)

Crawford J S, Potter S R 1984 Magnesium trisilicate mixture BP: its physical characteristics and effectiveness as a prophylactic. Anaesthesia 39 (in press)

Department of Health and Social Security 1979 Report on confidential enquiries into maternal deaths in England & Wales. Report on Health & Social Subjects No. 14.

Dewan D M, Wheeler A S, James F M, Floyd H M, Rhyne L 1982 Antacid anticholinergic regimens in patients undergoing elective Caesarean section. Canadian Anaesthetists' Society Journal 29: 27

Dow T G B, Brock-Utne J G, Rubin J, Welman S, Dimopoulos G E, Moshal M G 1978 Effect of atropine on the lower esophageal sphincter in late pregnancy. Obstetrics & Gynecology 51: 426

Gibbs C P, Schwartz D J, Wynne J W, Hood C I, Kuck E J 1979 Antacid pulmonary aspiration in the dog. Anesthesiology 51: 380

Gibbs C P, Spohr L, Schmidt D 1982 The effectiveness of sodium citrate as an antacid. Anesthesiology 57: 44

Holdsworth J D 1978 Relationship between stomach contents & analgesia in labour. British Journal of Anaesthesia 50: 1145

Holdsworth J D 1978 The place of apomorphine prior to obstetric analgesia. Journal of International Medical Research 6 (Suppl. 1): 26

Holdsworth J D, Johnson K, Mascall G, Roulston R G, Tomlinson P A 1980 Mixing of antacids with stomach contents. Anaesthesia 35: 641

Howard F A, Sharp D S 1973 Effect of metaclopramide on gastric emptying time during labour. British Medical Journal 1: 446

Johnson J R, Moore J, McCaughey W, Dundee J W, Howard P J, Tower W, McLean E 1983 Use of cimetidine as an oral antacid in obstetric anesthesia. Anesthesia and Analgesia 62: 720

Keating P J, Black J F, Watson D W 1978 Effects of glycopyrrolate & cimetidine on gastric volume & acidity in patients awaiting surgery. British Journal of Anaesthesia 50: 1247

Klein M D, Clahr J, Tamis A B, Solkow M L 1953 Maternal deaths caused by anesthesia in the Borough of the Bronx from 1940 to 1951. New York State Journal of Medicine 53: 2861

Lahiri S K, Thomas T A, Hodgson R M H 1973 Single dose antacid therapy for the prevention of Mendelson's syndrome. British Journal of Anaesthesia 45: 1143

McCaughey W, Howe J P, Moore J, Dundee J W 1981 Cimetidine in elective Caesarean section. Anaesthesia 36: 167

McGowan W A W 1979 Safety of cimetidine in obstetric patients. Journal of the Royal Society of Medicine 72: 902

Mendelson C L 1946 Aspiration of stomach contents into the lungs during obstetric anesthesia. American Journal of Obstetrics & Gynecology 52: 191

Morgan B M 1980 Maternal Death. Anaesthesia 35: 334

Pickering B G, Palahnuik R J, Cumming M 1980 Cimetidine premedication in elective Caesarean section. Canadian Anaesthetists' Society Journal 27: 33

Ranney B, Stanage W F 1975 Advantages of local anesthesia for Caesarean section. Obstetrics & Gynecology 45: 163

Smith G, Dalling R, Williams T I R 1978 Gastro-oesophageal pressure gradient changes produced by induction of anaesthesia & suxamethonium. British Journal of Anaesthesia 50: 1137

Stearns A B, Frederickson G C 1957 Promethazine hydrochloride for the control of nausea & vomiting during spinal anesthesia. Illinois Medical Journal 112: 267

Taylor G 1975 Acid pulmonary aspiration syndrome after antacids. British Journal of Anaesthesia 47: 615

Taylor G, Prys-Davis J 1966 Prophylactic use of antacids in the prevention of the acid-pulmonary-aspiration syndrome (Mendelson's syndrome) Lancet 1: 288

Tunstall M E 1976 Failed intubation drill (Summary). Anaesthesia 31: 850

Vandam L R 1965 Aspiration of gastric contents in the operative period. New England Journal of Medicine 273: 1206

Wheatley R G, Kallus F T, Reynolds R C, Giesecke A H 1979 Milk of magnesia is an effective pre-induction antacid in obstetric anesthesia. Anesthesiology 50: 514

5

Obstetric and non-obstetric complications affecting anaesthetic practice

Attention in this chapter is directed towards the impact upon anaesthetic practice of complications of obstetric origin and non-obstetric origin.

Complications of obstetric origin

It seems sensible to review these in the order in which they are likely to occur during the course of pregnancy.

Complications in early pregnancy

1. Spontaneous abortion

Almost the whole gamut of anaesthetic techniques is available for the provision of relief when the products of an aborted conceptus are to be evacuated.

General anaesthesia is probably the most commonly used method, but the poorest choice. The disadvantages include the customary six hour period of pre-operative starvation, the fairly unpleasant period of recovery and the slim, nonetheless real, dangers of complications associated with any general anaesthetic. The other major disadvantage is that it requires the services of an anaesthetist, which may not be readily available in some countries. Each of the other techniques to be described should be well within the competence of a reasonably-trained obstetrician. The only factor which favours the choice of general anaesthesia — other than an inability to provide any other form of anaesthesia — is the emotional state of the patient. If she is extremely upset because of her failed pregnancy, kindness dictates that she should be asleep during the operation.

Hypoaesthesia is a technique of subliminal general anaesthesia which has long been advocated in several situations (Crawford 1958a). It consists of an intravenous injection of a mixture containing a narcotic analgesic and a tranquilliser. The specific identity of each drug is not of great importance. Pethidine 100 mg plus promazine 50 mg has been used (Crawford 1958b) as has morphia plus promazine (Whitney 1966); diazepam 10 mg could be substituted for promazine in combination with pethidine. The drugs must be well diluted, preferably to a volume of 20 ml, and injected slowly. In the unlikely event that the patient complains of some discomfort during the operation, she should be encouraged to breathe from one of the four approved intermittent inhalational apparatuses described earlier. It would be unusual if the cervical os were to be resistant to the introduction of instruments, but if such is the case, two inhalations of salbutamol from a standard Ventolin inhaler will provide the required relaxation. *Hypoaesthesia should not be provided whilst the patient is either hypotensive or hypovolaemic.*

Paracervical block appears not to have found favour, although it would seem to be a reasonable choice. There is no fetus to be placed in jeopardy, sensation from the uterus (with the possible exception of the fundus) is obtunded, and the obstetrician is well-conversant with the anatomical features of the block-site. If the rule of 'aspiration before injection' is strictly followed, and the dose is limited to 10 ml of one per cent lignocaine (plain) on each side, the attendant complications should be of an extremely low order.

Extra-dural block specifically for this operation could probably be categorised as a virtuoso performance, having little relevance to routine clinical practice. However, a single-shot caudal block would be a reasonable choice. In this context it must be borne in mind that the block requires to be extended cephalad to T10, and that as the patient is not pregnant the available capacity of her extra-dural space is greater than it would be if she were at term. Thus the volume of local anaesthetic required is likely to be 25–30 ml, and the patient should lie supine for 10–15 minutes after the injection so that her thoraco-lumbar lordosis prevents any untoward spread beyond the lower thoracic roots. Bupivacaine would be a poor choice of local anaesthetic, because only a brief duration of analgesia is required. Chloroprocaine would be the drug of choice, were it to become available in the U.K., but currently one per cent lignocaine (plain) is the recommended agent.

Spinal block in cases of evacuation of retained products of conception is becoming increasingly popular, and is currently the method of choice in the Birmingham Maternity Hospital. This approach is an option in other situations to be discussed in this Chapter, and it seems appropriate to describe the technique here.

Spinal block technique

This discussion has relevance only to the conduct of cases in which the block is not required to be extended further cephalad than T10; (its application in caesarean section has been referred to in the preceding Chapter.) The local anaesthetic solutions used are therefore hyperbaric — i.e., their specific gravity is greater than is that of cerebrospinal fluid (c.s.f.); the extent of spread within the c.s.f. is thus governed predominantly by the influence of gravity. Hyperbaricity is achieved by the inclusion of dextrose in a concentration of five or six per cent in the solution.

Three local anaesthetics for spinal analgesia have been available in the U.K. to a varying extent.

These are (i) heavy Nupercaine (cinchocaine) as 2.5 mg of the drug per 1 ml of 5 per cent dextrose; (ii) 5 per cent lignocaine in 7.5 per cent dextrose; (iii) 5 per cent prilocaine in 6 per cent dextrose. Of these, the first has been somewhat erratically available because of manufacturing difficulties and the last was withdrawn in 1978 because of stability problems. Lignocaine has not received the seal of approval for use as a spinal anaesthetic, from the Committee of Safety of Drugs and is not commercially available. However, it can be dispensed by the Department of Pharmacy in any large hospital, or group of hospitals, and there should be no difficulty in obtaining a supply. The only distinguishing feature worth noting amongst the three drugs is their respective duration of action. Total recovery from sensory block after Nupercaine takes 10 hours, after prilocaine 4 hours and after lignocaine 2 hours. However the duration of the operative procedures under consideration is briefer than the shortest of these periods of drug effect.

An isobaric solution of 0.5 per cent bupivacaine is achieving increasing popularity for spinal analgesia in this country, but its use in obstetric practice here has not been well-documented. Its duration of effective action lies between 3 and 5 hours.

The essential immediate preliminaries to the initiation of a spinal block are: (i) the patient's blood pressure must be measured and recorded; (ii) an intravenous infusion must be in progress.

The anaesthetic solution spreads through the c.s.f. mainly in response to gravity, and the majority of the injected drug is rapidly fixed by elements of nervous tissue. Therefore, it is preferable to conduct a spinal block with the patient in the sitting position. She sits sideways on the operating table or delivery bed, with her legs hanging over the side and an assistant supporting her. The patient's back should be bowed as much as possible and her vertebral column should be vertical with respect to the bed or table. The skin is prepared with the usual antiseptic solution, and a reasonably wide lumbar interspace is defined by palpation (the level of the iliac crests provides a guide to the space beween the second and third or third and fourth lumbar spines). Local infiltration of the skin is not required because the spinal needle is of fine gauge, usually a 25-gauge or finer. It may be introduced via a 23-gauge needle which has been advanced as far as the ligamentum flavum — this manoeuvre is advisable if a 26 or 27-gauge spinal needle is to be used, because of the great flexibility of these fine instruments.

Penetration of the dura will frequently be recognised by a snapping sensation, but just as often will be assumed to have been achieved because of the depth to which the needle has been advanced (provided that the advance has been made at absolute right-angles to the transverse plane of the back and with a slight cephalad angulation to steer it between the spinous processes). When the stilette is withdrawn c.s.f, might appear within the needle, but this is by no means invariable, because the bore of the chosen needle may be too narrow. More frequently, c.s.f. can be aspirated into an attached 2 ml syringe. Quite often, however, such direct evidence of penetration of the dura is not obtained, and reliance is placed upon the 'feel' of the procedure and upon lack of resistance to injection of the local anaesthetic solution.

The volume of solution injected is usually the same (1.25 ml) whichever of the three local anaesthetics referred to is used, but a particularly large patient may require 1.5 ml. The solution is injected during a timed period 10 seconds, and as soon as the injection is complete, the needle is withdrawn, the patient is told to sit upright and a clean gauze swab is applied to the injection site. The length of time the patient remains sitting depends upon how high a block is required. If analgesia extending to T10 is needed, as for an evacuation of retained products, the period should be 5 seconds. If analgesia of only the perineum is required, the patient should remain upright for 15 seconds. As soon as the determined period has elapsed, the patient should be helped rapidly to lie supine with her head and shoulders on pillows, and tilted laterally on a wedge if she is still pregnant. The blood pressure is taken again and subsequently at 5 minute intervals during the next 20 minutes. The block will be effective within 3–5 minutes and the patient may then be placed into the lithotomy position.

The outstanding complication of spinal analgesia is headache. As with the headache resulting from an inadvertent dural tap, this is postural in character and may persist for as long a six days if untreated. The incidence is, to some extent, dependant upon the gauge of the needle with which the dura was pierced, although in our experience (Crawford 1979) there had been little difference between 23 and 25-gauge. *The incidence of headache in obstetric anaesthetic practice appears to be considerably higher than that usually quoted for the whole of anaesthetic practice.* This might reflect the fluid shifts which typically occur in the post-partum period, and the fact that obstetric patients are neither required nor desire to remain in bed for several days after the anaesthetic. In our series of 443 spinals (Crawford 1979) the percentage incidence of headache related to the operative procedure was roughly as follows:

Vaginal delivery	16%
Retained placenta	21%
'Other'	13%

'Other' operations included a considerable number of cases of evacuation of retained products, and as these were virtually non-pregnant patients, this might explain their lower incidence of headache. The headache can be rapidly and permanently cured by the provision of an epidural blood patch. If the patient declines the offer of this therapy, she should be encouraged to rest as much as possible, and be assured that the headache will clear spontaneously on the sixth day. A tightly-applied abdominal binder is frequently of help in reducing the severity of the headache, presumably because it causes engorgement of the epidural veins, secondary to increasing intra-abdominal pressure, and thereby reduces the rate of outflow of c.s.f. through the dural puncture.

If the spinal has been given with scrupulous attention to the details outlined, other complications should be extremely rare. A high spinal block, involving the mid and upper thoracic roots, is a potential hazard which has achieved undue notoriety. Unless the spinal has been grossly mismanaged, this infrequent occurrence need occasion no great alarm. A fall in blood pressure might result, and this can be reversed by the rapid infusion of crystalloid solution intravenously; very rarely will a vasopressor be required. If there is a degree of respiratory embarrassment, oxygen should be supplied via a mask; rarely, ventilatory support via a mask or an endotracheal tube may be indicated.

Complications of this order are rarities. However, detailing them serves to draw attention to the major contra-indications to providing a spinal block. A spinal should not be given if the equipment necessary to provide the appropriate resuscitation — and a clinician who is well conversant with its application — is not immediately available. A spinal must not be provided for a patient who is hypotensive or hypovolaemic.

2. Termination of a mid-trimester pregnancy

Continuous lumbar epidural block is ideally suited to the care of the patient who undergoes a mid-trimester termination of pregnancy. The process of the termination, usually initiated by the use of prostaglandins, is frequently prolonged, potentially painful and may be concluded by exploration and evacuation of the uterine cavity. If the facilities for providing an epidural are available, there is no justification for denying them. The block should be as extensive as for term labour. Sympathy dictates that the patient should also be given a tranquilliser (diazepam 5 mg intravenously or orally) at appropriate intervals throughout her labour.

3. Insertion of a Shirodkhar suture

General anaesthesia is a poor choice for this operation, unless the patient insists upon being asleep, or there is a deficiency of anaesthetic expertise available to provide a regional block. The restlessness which is associated with emergence from a general anaesthetic, with its attendant likelihood of vomiting, poses an unwelcome challenge. A spinal block may be used but a better choice would be continuous lumbar epidural block. The advantages of an epidural are that it is not associated with a significant incidence of post-anaesthetic headache and it can be maintained for an indefinite period post-operatively.

Intermittent pain is experienced by some patients during the first 24 hours after encirclage of the cervix, and a continuous epidural will guard against this. In many obstetric units a narcotic analgesic is prescribed to ease pain and in the belief that such medication will help to 'dampen down' any threatening uterine activity. The grounds for this belief are somewhat dubious, as noted in a preceding chapter, but if there is a basis of truth in it, then an epidural block will be equally as effective. An added advantage is that the nausea, and even vomiting, plus general unease of the patient which occur during repetitive administration of narcotics will not be evidenced by an epidural.

Complications in late pregnancy

1. Pre-eclamptic toxaemia

The anaesthetist has a considerable role to play in the collaborative care of the patient with moderate or severe pre-eclampsia (PET). If the condition of the patient deteriorates, or if she is admitted to hospital with moderate or severe PET, she needs intensive care, and the cooperation of an informed obstetric anaesthetist should be available.

Increasingly, the opinion is hardening that prompt delivery is likely to offer the best chance of perinatal survival and to limit maternal morbidity. However, if the condition of the fetus appears to be satisfactory, and the mother is not in labour, an effort may first be made to reduce the blood pressure to a tolerable level using either methyldopa, labetolol or hydralazine. The latter is likely to be the drug of choice for the acute situation in most centres, as its site of action is predominantly on the peripheral vasculature. It may be given intravenously (20 mg) as a loading dose, and subsequently by mouth; it is also advisable to prescribe diazepam (5 mg orally thrice daily) to reduce the patient's anxiety and raise her 'convulsion threshold'. If these measures stabilise the patient's condition, and she is not in labour, further urgent action is not required.

The labouring patient with moderate or severe PET must be guarded against a rise in blood pressure or an abrupt and severe fall because vaso-motor tone may be particularly sensitive to the pressor effect of catecholamines (Talledo et al 1968), making her blood pressure labile. Thus analgesia is an essential component of therapy. Also, anti-hypertensive therapy will be continued in order to maintain the blood pressure at the previously established level. Each of these requirements can be met by providing an epidural block sufficiently extensive to induce considerable loss of vasomotor tone (Moir et al 1972). I prefer not to use epidural block for this dual purpose, because it does not provide a sufficiently fine control of blood pressure. I prefer to use the epidural primarily to provide analgesia, and to regulate blood pressure by means of hydralazine delivered intravenously with the aid of a pump. The epidural will undoubtedly cause some reduction of blood pressure; in order to avoid episodes of unacceptable lowering of the pressure it is essential that the rate of infusion of hydralazine be reduced during the few minutes before initiation of the block, and before each top-up dose is given. This will allow for restabilisation following induction or extension of vasodilatation.

It should by now be well understood that ergometrine must not be given to a pre-eclamptic mother except as the penultimate resort in the treatment of postpartum uterine hypotonia. Eclampsia presenting de novo after delivery is a well known entity, and many of these cases encountered in the past might have been triggered by ergometrine.

Two factors which are of prime importance to the consideration of the treatment of PET have yet to be discussed; hypovolaemia and placental perfusion.

Hypovolaemia

It is still not widely appreciated that, despite the characteristic oedema associated with PET, the patient has a reduced circulating blood volume. The hypovolaemia is, in part, due to the increased permeability of capillary walls, and a disparity in albumin concentration between the intravascular and extravascular fluid compartments. In pre-eclampsia the serum albumin concentration is even lower than that in normal pregnancy, whereas the mass of extravascular albumin is the same (Henshall 1979). Thus, the osmotic gradient favours the passage of fluid out of the vascular system.

The presence of hypovolaemia has important implications in the treatment of hypertension and in the induction of vaso-dilatation with a regional block. In the normotensive subject, if vascular capacitance is increased in the presence of hypovolaemia, a severe fall in blood pressure is likely to result; this classically occurs in the mismanagement of a patient in shock. For the same reason, an epidural block of an extent appropriate to providing analgesia in labour is very much more likely to cause severe hypotension in a hypovolaemic pre-eclamptic patient, than is the same block given to a normotensive patient. It is essential to the proper care of the pre-eclamptic patient to correct, at least in good part, her hypovolaemia before an epidural is initiated; this is best attained by the intravenous infusion of a crystalloid solution.

Placental perfusion

It has for long been assumed that placental perfusion is reduced in pre-eclampsia. This assumption has been verified by a series of investigations of intervillous blood flow assessed by the clearance rate of ^{133}Xe (Kaar et al 1980). These workers have demonstrated that severe PET is associated with a highly significant reduction of intervillous blood flow relative to that found during normal pregnancy. It has also been shown that although a segmental epidural block (Chapter 2) does not lead to a significant increase in intervillous blood flow in PET (Jouppila et al 1979) a full block extending caudally from T10 does cause such an increase (Jouppila et al 1982). Thus the provision of an epidural should benefit the fetus by increasing placental perfusion.

Some workers have argued that in patients with PET reducing blood pressure may be unhelpful because the pressure may be necessary for good placental perfusion. One response to those who have such reservations has just been provided. The other response rests upon an understanding of the dynamics of the situation. In the normotensive patient the utero-placental vessels spurt intermittently (Martin et al 1964, Power et al 1967), periods of complete closure alternating with periods of full dilatation. The supply of arterialised maternal blood to the placental site is *pressure dependant* and a sustained reduction of maternal blood pressure would diminish the efficiency of intervillous blood flow. In the hypertensive patient, however, the utero-placental vessels are, in common with the remainder of the peripheral vasculature, partially constricted and circulation through the placental bed is predominantly *flow dependant*.

The genesis of this distinction lies early in the maternal history of pre-eclampsia. Secondary invasion by trophoblast which, under normal circumstances takes place at about 16 weeks gestation, destroys the musculo-elastic wall of the spiral arteries, and its attendant vaso-motor nerve supply. These end-arteries, which open funnel-like into the intervillous space, thereafter have a fibrous coat which is not responsive to neuro-humoral stimuli. In the mother who is destined to develop the clinically-evident syndrome of pre-eclampsia this secondary invasion does not occur, and the spiral arteries retain their musculo-elastic wall together with its nerve supply. Thus the vessels which supply the intervillous space will share the same response as those exhibited by the remainder of the mother's peripheral vasculature. Furthermore, as has been noted, in pre-eclampsia these vessels are particularly sensitive to the vaso-constrictor action of catecholamines, and will therefore exhibit hypertonicity throughout much of the final trimester. An anti-hypertensive agent will, by reducing vascular tone, improve perfusion of the intervillous space. An epidural given for labour and delivery exerts a beneficial effect of even wider scope. It blocks the vaso-motor nerves which supply the spiral arteries, rendering them maximally dilated, and by preventing pain and apprehension it averts the increased outpouring of catecholamines which is otherwise a characteristic of labour.

Despite the above factors, it cannot be claimed that an epidural (or anti-hypertensive therapy) offers the opportunity of returning intervillous blood flow, and hence feto-maternal exchange in the pre-eclamptic, to normality. Neither therapy will alleviate the obstruction due to deposition of fibrin over the external aspects of the fetal villi or that caused by platelet aggregation in the micro-circulation of the placenta (Inglis et al 1982).

Two subsidiary effects of an epidural given to a patient with PET may be beneficial. The sympathetic nerve supply to the kidneys and the suprarenals is supplied from the nerve roots T10–11; an epidural block of the advocated extent might increase renal blood flow and reduce the rate of secretion of catecholamines by the suprarenal glands.

This form of management cannot be fully pursued if the mother has a *coagulation defect*. An epidural block must not be initiated unless very recent evidence of a normal 'coagulation profile' has been obtained. If the laboratory report suggests that bleeding and clotting times are prolonged beyond the normal range, some other form of analgesia must be provided.

It is in this situation that we have found the Cardiff Palliator to be of considerable benefit (Harper et al 1983). This apparatus permits the labouring woman to self-administer pethidine intravenously in bolus quantities, of pre-determined amount, at intervals whose minimum duration are also pre-set.

In the previous edition of this book it is stated that regional analgesia is not advisable for caesarean section of a pre-eclamptic mother. That statement requires modification. If the mother is severely pre-eclamptic, possibly hyper-reflexic, or with evidence of coagulopathy, general anaesthesia is virtually mandatory. For the mother who has received considerable anti-convulsant therapy, and is therefore likely to be restless if operated upon whilst awake, it would be unwise to provide an epidural for her section. However, the increasing tendency to delivery by section before pre-eclampsia develops to such a degree of severity has allowed us, as well as anaesthetists in other well-experienced units, to offer mothers with mild or moderate pre-eclampsia an epidural for either elective or emergency section.

The technique of general anaesthesia does not differ from that detailed in the previous Chapter, with one exception: a transparent, plastic endotracheal tube with a high volume low pressure cuff should be used because the patient should be maintained on a ventilator with humidification for at least six hours after the end of the operation. Use of this tube reduces the likelihood of resultant laryngotracheal trauma; Seager & Macdonald (1980) have reported that laryngeal oedema may accompany pre-eclampsia and this should spur the anaesthetist to extra care in the process of intubation. It is well-recognised that endotracheal intubation provokes a rise of blood pressure, and it has been advocated that in severe PET this hypertensive response should be prevented by an intravenous infusion of nitroglycerine, starting a few minutes before induction and continuing until delivery (Snyder et al 1979). The results of this form of management in a reasonably large series have not yet been published.

2. Eclampsia

The patient who is admitted in eclampsia, or who unexpectedly fits whilst under care, requires immediate anti-convulsant therapy and ventilatory support. Oxygen should be given via a face-mask and suction made immediately available. Anaesthesia is induced with either thiopentone (250 mg) or diazepam (20 mg). Suxamethonium (100 mg) is then given intravenously and an endotracheal tube passed.

We have now considered three situations; severe pre-eclampsia in a labouring patient; fulminating pre-eclampsia and eclampsia. In each instance delivery by caesarean section might be included within the total management. These three situations converge in some respects to a final common point — the need for highly intensive care. Labour itself requires intensive care, while moderate or severe pre-eclampsia demands a greater intensity of supervision.

Intensive care facilities

There should be a room designated for the care of high-risk patients in the delivery suite of every obstetric unit which is well enough staffed and equipped to care for such mothers. Such a room should be furnished with all the equipment likely to be required for the treatment and monitoring of patients with severe pre-eclampsia or other serious complications. In the event of an emergency, time must not be wasted searching for disposable items, containers for laboratory samples and the like. Of equal or greater importance is a protocol of management devised and agreed upon by all senior medical and nursing staff. Junior members of staff should be familiarised with this protocol when they start their tour of duty so that they can take informed action without hesitation, and without the delay incumbent upon trying to contact senior colleagues for urgent advice. All items of equipment must be left in a state of readiness, and this demands regular weekly inspections, as well as trials of apparatus, by a responsible member of the staff.

Monitoring equipment

The monitoring requirements include the following:

a. An intra-uterine pressure and fetal heart rate monitor;

b. A blood pressure monitor. During the acute phase of the illness the patient's blood pressure should be recorded at 15–20 minute intervals; the use of a standard sphygmomanometer for this is time consuming for the midwifery staff, disturbing for the patient, of dubious reliability and prone to across-observer error. It is preferable to use an automated blood pressure recorder. An intra-arterial monitor would be better still, but the hazards associated with its occasional use in a unit whose medical and nursing staff are not fully conversant with the technique probably mitigate against the choice.

c. A scrupulously kept fluid balance chart. To this end it is highly advisable that an in-dwelling urinary catheter be inserted at the earliest convenient time. Samples of urine must be submitted daily for estimation of protein concentration.

d. The acid-base values and oxygen tension in samples of arterial blood should be assessed at least once each day during the acute phase. These estimations should be repeated more frequently during the immediate post-operative period, and if the patient is on a ventilator.

e. A daily platelet count is necessary and if the count is low or is falling, a series of tests to determine the patient's coagulation status should be obtained.

f. A full blood count, serum electrolytes, serum protein concentrations, blood urea, creatinine and uric acid should be determined daily.

g. The advisability of setting up a central venous pressure (c.v.p.) line is a matter for clincial judgement. If the recordings are reliable, they will be of considerable help in making decisions about the volumes of intravenous fluids which can be rapidly and safely given, but there is a danger associated with the practice. *It will occasionally happen that the wall of a major vessel is penetrated during the establishment of a c.v.p. line.* Under most circumstances, this causes little or no harm. However, if there is a coagulopathy, or if one develops before the breach in the vessel wall has been sealed, serious haemorrhage can occur into the thoracic cavity. The decision to monitor the c.v.p. is therefore a matter of balanced clinical judgement, but a line must not be inserted unless there is evidence that the coagulation factors are within normal limits.

h. A plain X-ray of the chest should be obtained at a convenient time post-operatively, and repeated each day during the acute phase of the patient's illness.

Fundamentals of intensive treatment

a. Drug management

The fundamental bases of treatment are anti-hypertensive therapy and anti-convulsant therapy. The current anti-hypertensive agent of choice is hydralazine; an excellent review of anti-hypertensive drugs which may be considered in the treatment of PET has been published by Berkowitz (1980). Hydralazine should be given by pump infusion and my own practice is also to infuse diazepam as the anti-convulsant of choice. A 50 ml syringe containing 40 mg of diazepam is a convenient method. Chlormethiazole is an alternative choice of anti-convulsant, but this must of necessity be given by drip infusion, which in the long-term care of patients, is open to accidents of under- or over-dosage. On a very few occasions we have found diazepam to be ineffective in suitably reducing the patient's irritability, and substituting chlormethiazole has proved to be satisfactory.

The appropriate rate of administration of each of these drugs is a matter of clinical judgement concerning the individual patient. In respect to the anti-hypertensive, the objective should be to maintain the systolic blood pressure between 120–150 mmHg. The anti-convulsant dosage should be such as to prevent any restlessness and overt irritability of the patient whilst avoiding, if possible, profound c.n.s. depression. An element of depression is inherent in the therapy and there should be no reluctance to maintain or initiate ventilatory support particularly during the immediate post-operative period.

The phase of recovery from general anaesthesia is characteristically one of restlessness and considerable physiological imbalance. The gap occurring between recovery from the anaesthetic and institution of anti-convulsant therapy is potentially hazardous; it is most advisable to bridge this with the aid of controlled ventilation. Until recently it has been foreign to obstetric practice to have an unanaesthetised patient ventilated in a delivery suite. But the general tenets of intensive care condemn a situation in which a heavily sedated patient is allowed to be nursed without an assured airway.

b. Ventilatory care

The ventilator should be relatively unsophisticated as, in general, midwives are not conversant with this aspect of patient care; I have chosen to use a Cape ventilator. The inspired gas mixture must be humidified adequately and although ventilation with air might prove to be satisfactory, blood gas analyses during the acute phase will usually reveal the need to provide additional oxygen. It has been demonstrated that a slight but not significant lowering of arterial oxygen tension is associated with severe PET, indicative of a degree of pulmonary ventilation-perfusion imbalance (Templeton & Kelman 1977). It is probable that this is mainly due to microemboli in the pulmonary circulation (Birmingham Eclampsia Study Group 1971).

c. Physiotherapy

Whether or not the patient is receiving ventilatory support, she will require the services of a physiotherapist. It is important that for 15 minutes before each episode of chest physiotherapy (which should be conducted at least twice daily) the rate of infusion of diazepam should be increased lest the stimulation provokes a hypertensive response and possibly an eclamptic fit.

d. A naso-gastric tube

This should invariably be in place throughout the acute phase of the illness, and 15 ml magnesium trisilicate mixture BPC injected through it every two hours.

e. Analgesia

It is important to bear in mind that diazepam is not an analgesic. If the patient has not been given an epidural block, a narcotic analgesic should be given at appropriate intervals during the first 24–48 hours after delivery by caesarean section.

f. Coagulation problems

A severe coagulation defect, with haemorrhage and evidence of widespread disseminated intravascular coagulation, demands urgent management. It would be inappropriate to discuss here the available options, each situation demanding a tailored regimen preferably arrived at with the help of a haematologist. If a very low, or rapidly falling platelet count is the only manifestation of the disease, consideration should be given to the administration of a concentrated preparation of fresh platelets.

g. Fluid therapy and balance

This is one of the most important yet generally least well understood items in the care of the severely pre-eclamptic patient. As has already been emphasised, hypovolaemia is a characteristic of pre-eclampsia, and it is likely that the degree of reduction in the

142

circulating blood volume correlates directly with the severity of the disease. To some extent, the hypertension can be considered as being compensatory, though such a view is not necessarily correct; however, it helps to bring into sharper focus the juxtaposition of hypovolaemia and peripheral vasoconstriction. This combination results in a diminished perfusion of tissues, including the utero-placental complex and the kidneys. Thus, despite the fact that the patient is oedematous due to the imbalance between intravascular and extracellular concentrations of albumin, *fluids must be given and not withheld*; this holds true irrespective of the urinary output. Indeed, the more severe the degree of oliguria the more urgent is the need to infuse fluid intravenously, as the reduction in renal excretion reflects hypoperfusion of the kidneys, which, if allowed to persist for long, can lead to irreversible renal damage.

An even greater folly than a strict limitation of fluid replenishment is to administer a diuretic. This latter error of management will succeed only in reducing still further her circulating blood volume, possibly resulting in an episode of severe hypotension, and making her condition more parlous. Thiazide diuretics have the added danger of inducing acute, and occasionally fatal, pancreatitis. If the liberal administration of fluids is correctly managed, there is no need for the clinician to be concerned if a protracted period of oliguria occurs; this is especially so in patients who have been delivered by caesarean section. Normally there is a reduction in urinary output throughout the first six hours post-operatively, reflecting the response to stress and general anaesthesia. Severe PET and eclampsia merely compound the oliguria. It has not been unusual in our practice for a marked diuresis to be delayed for 36–48 hours post-operatively.

The intravenously infused fluid should be a crystalloid solution (Hartmann's or Ringer-Lactate) interspersed with 5 per cent dextrose in the relation of three bottles to one respectively. Preferably this regimen should be monitored by reference to the central venous pressure. The c.v.p. is usually very low in severe PET, reflective of the hypovolaemia. The objective of fluid therapy is to increase the c.v.p. to 6–10 cm water. The major complication of such fluid therapy is to overload the patient and cause consequent pulmonary oedema. If the c.v.p. is not monitored, considerable attention must be paid to frequent auscultation of the dependent areas of the lungs. If pulmonary oedema should develop, a diuretic must be administered; the drug of choice is mannitol. While cerebral oedema is unlikely to result from excessive fluid administration it can occur during PET and is yet another manifestation of the extracellular accumulation of fluid. Treatment is advisable if there is evidence of considerable cerebral oedema; dexamethasone should be administered, and if the patient is being ventilated, the minute volume should be increased to reduce the arterial carbon dioxide tension and thus induce a modicum of cerebral vasoconstriction.

An additional form of therapy has attracted international attention but little has yet been published. This consists of administering aliquots of human plasma protein fraction (PPF) intravenously. The objective is to increase the intravascular concentration of protein and thereby to redress the balance of colloid osmotic pressures across the capillary endothelium and hence maintain intravascular volume. The aliquots dispensed nationally by the Blood Transfusion Service consist of 400 ml of PPF (containing 17.2–18.0 g protein). These are given at intervals of about 8 hours. As has been demonstrated (Joyce et al 1979) this results in an impressive rise of c.v.p. to the normal range, an amelioration of the hypertension and a consequent initiation of a diuresis. It is unlikely that more than three aliquots (or 1200 ml) will be required over 24 hours. A further finding reported by Joyce and his colleagues (1979) was that, prior to the start of protein therapy, there was a considerable disparity between the central haematocrit obtained by sampling from the c.v.p. line, and the haematocrit of peripheral blood. This disparity had been reduced to within 1 per cent, the normal relation between the two values, when treatment was completed. The major complication of this therapy is pulmonary oedema, and c.v.p. monitoring is therefore highly advisable. There is, however, some prospect that monitoring may be effectively performed by frequent estimations of the colloid oncotic pressure of the patient's plasma, though present colloid osmometers are temperamental machines. The intravenous administration of dextran instead of PPF has been reported to be of value in this situation (Sehgal & Hitt 1980).

h. Weaning

The gradual weaning of the patient from the major items of therapy, namely the ventilator and anti-hypertensive and anti-convulsant drugs, is a matter of clinical skill and judgement; precipitate withdrawal of any of these is to be avoided. A somewhat overextended period of therapy is preferable to discontinuing too early. Ventilator therapy should be maintained until the patient is reasonably alert and virtually removes her endotracheal tube with coordination and intelligent purpose. We have very rarely found it necessary to maintain these patients on skeletal muscle relaxants in order to facilitate ventilation, so the appropriate time for extubation is reasonably well apparent.

The rate of the hydralazine infusion is reduced in accord with the trend of falling blood pressure. It may be necessary on occasion to reverse this procedure, as often the blood pressure will tend to increase again as the mother's level of consciousness lightens and she becomes more aware of discomfort. The general trend, however, is that hydralazine is unlikely to be required for longer than 3-4 days. It is advisable to substitute methyldopa for hydralazine when the rate of infusion of the latter approaches zero, and to maintain therapy with methyldopa for several days subsequently.

The appropriate rate of weaning from anti-convulsant coverage provides the most difficult challenge. The appearance of maternal distress, or of a 'spike' of blood pressure, should prompt an increase in the rate of infusion of diazepam. After a period of quiescence the rate of infusion can be slowly and gradually reduced, but the period of weaning is more likely to be a matter of days rather than hours.

There should be no imposed restriction on the food provided for the patient upon her recovery from the acute phase. Most of our patients are hungry when they emerge from the effects of the diazepam, or are released from the ventilator. They avidly eat the jelly and ice-cream (the latter usually fortified with additional calories and vitamins) which is first offered to them, and rapidly progress to taking a substantial diet rich in protein, calories and vitamins. If the acute phase of the illness is unusually protracted, it is advisable to provide quantities of concentrates such as Casilan via the gastric tube.

Complications during labour and delivery

1. Presence of a uterine scar

A uterine scar must occasion increased vigilance, but not cause anxiety of a degree that will distort clinical judgement. Despite the deeply-engrained opinion of many obstetricians lacking personal experience of this situation, a continuous epidural block is indicated, rather than contraindicated, in the care of a labouring patient who has been delivered previously by caesarean section or who has had a myomectomy. The declared fear is that the regional block will prevent the appreciation of pain due to an impending or actual scar rupture but such is not the case. Pain is a relatively infrequent manifestation of impending or actual scar rupture; a change in the pattern of uterine contractions, evidence of fetal distress and fresh vaginal bleeding provide evidence much more frequently. If pain does occur as a feature of this complication it will break through the sensory block of an epidural (Crawford 1976). Indeed, an epidural block which effectively prevents the pain of a uterine contraction will, in the event of an impending rupture, still allow tenderness to palpation over the site of the scar to be elicited. The mother will usually complain of persistent pain well localised to the point of impending or actual rupture. Thus an effective epidural relieves the obstetrician of the anxiety associated with trying to decide whether the pain complained of by his patient is the pain of labour or the pain of scar dehiscence.

I have not had cause for regret in the administration of a continuous epidural block for the labour of more than 500 patients who had previously been delivered by caesarean section. The aphorism could be that, if the obstetrician is content to allow his patient to labour, the anaesthetist is more than willing to provide her with an epidural.

2. Delivery with forceps or ventouse

The point has been made previously that if the mother has had an epidural for labour she can, with ease and gentleness, be delivered with the aid of forceps or the ventouse. It has also been stressed that the obstetrician should resist the temptation to effect the delivery too early.

If an epidural is not in progress, and the decision is made that instrumental delivery of an infant presenting by the vertex is necessary, *the first choice of anaesthesia is a spinal block*. The only exceptions to this are: (i) the absence of anyone competent to administer a spinal; (ii) the presenting part is so low on the perineum that a simple lift-out forceps can be conducted after infiltration of the proposed line of the episiotomy with local anaesthetic solution.

The spinal is administered as described previously. The objective is to block the emergent spinal roots from T10 to S5, so that after the local anaesthetic agent has been injected into the c.s.f., the patient should sit bolt upright for 5 seconds, and then be rapidly swung to the horizontal position with left lateral tilt to avoid aorto-caval compression. The blood pressure should be monitored at 5 minute intervals during the subsequent 20 minutes, and the upper limit of sensory loss assessed. The mother may be placed into the lithotomy position, with lateral tilt in less than 5 minutes following injection of the local anaesthetic. Excellent analgesia and profound relaxation of the pelvic floor will result. The bearing-down sensation will not be experienced but the mother will be able to co-operate when requested to push with contractions. Therefore, in the absence of fetal distress, and the need for urgent delivery, the opportunity allows further descent of the presenting part in order to reduce the trauma associated with delivery.

Pudendal block is the time-honoured alternative technique of anaesthesia. If executed correctly — a rather rare event in most obstetric units according to Scudamore & Yates (1966) — it provides reasonable relief from the pain of a low forceps delivery. If rotation of the fetal head is part of the procedure, or if it is a mid-forceps delivery, the quality of analgesia provided by a pudendal block is relatively poor. *In cases of outlet forceps delivery, a pudendal block, whether administered using the transvaginal route or the transperineal route, affords no advantage over a generous infiltration of the perineum with local anaesthetic.*

Simple observation will convince any practitioner of the advantage of a spinal over a pudendal block (Hutchins 1980). As soon as the spinal has been induced the mother will relax and her face will become a picture of relief and satisfaction. She will enjoy her delivery, conducted by an obstetrician untrammelled by the anxieties associated with a squirming patient who bears down uncontrollably and complains of discomfort or pain. The pudendal rarely offers the latter advantages and must, therefore, encompass greater potential hazard to the fetus.

3. Vaginal delivery of breech presentation, multiple pregnancy and the immature or low birthweight infant

These categories of delivery are grouped together because they make similar demands upon the obstetric anaesthetist. The major dangers to infants in these situations are birth trauma and a prolonged period of intra-uterine asphyxia during the second-stage and delivery. The outstanding cause of trauma is a poorly controlled delivery of a mother who is bearing down involuntarily and whose pelvic floor is tense or poorly relaxed. The overwhelming evidence presented during recent years is that regional block provides the greatest defence against these hazards (Crawford 1974, Crawford 1975, James et al 1977, Jaschevatzky et al 1977, Weeks et al 1977, Gullestad & Sagan 1977, Breeson et al 1978, De Crespigny & Pepperell 1979, Jarvis & Whitefield 1981). The objectives of the regional block are to relieve pain, to relax the pelvic floor and completely to abolish the bearing-down reflex. Satisfaction of this triad of aims permits the obstetrician to accomplish an unhurried, gently-assisted delivery. There can be no doubting that this results in a significant reduction in the hazard of intra-cranial haemorrhage, a characteristic associated with these cases and particularly, with light for dates infants. It must be emphasised that there is no justification for hurrying the delivery process in the absence of convincing evidence of fetal distress.

In a breech delivery, whether of a singleton or a twin, the requirement to conduct a breech extraction is not increased by the use of this technique of anaesthesia. If an epidural block is in progress when the second-stage approaches, it will be the analgesic technique of choice for the delivery. If a patient in this category presents late in labour and there is insufficient time to initiate a satisfactory epidural block, spinal analgesia must be the technique of choice.

The results of a recent study, completed but not yet reported, strongly suggest that when vaginal delivery is conducted under an epidural, the incidence of a second twin being in a better condition, both clinically and biochemically, is no less than that of a first twin being the better. This contrasts with the immediate outcome of twin deliveries conducted without regional analgesia, in which almost invariably the second twin is in either a worse, or no better, condition than its sibling. The mean interval between deliveries was virtually the same in both series.

Intra-uterine asphyxia is most likely to occur as a result of aorto-caval compression in the patients under discussion. They are likely to be in the lithotomy position for a considerable length of time before delivery is accomplished and must be effectively tilted — preferably to the left — throughout this period. It was the failure to appreciate this requirement in years gone by, which promoted the criticism of the use of regional block for this type of delivery.

An additional measure which might be of benefit is to encourage the mother to breathe from a source of supplemental oxygen throughout the second-stage, especially for the delivery of the second twin whose placental site is contracted following delivery of the first twin.

No reference has been made to the provision of general anaesthesia in these cases and the omission is no accident. A requirement to give a general anaesthetic for vaginal delivery must, with few exceptions, be considered a failure of obstetric or anaesthetic organisation and care. The oustanding exception is when a trial of forceps is to be undertaken upon a mother who does not have an epidural block in progress and who might require to be delivered urgently by caesarean section, if it becomes evident that vaginal delivery cannot be safely accomplished.

Maternal morbidity and mortality associated with general anaesthesia is significantly greater than that associated with regional analgesia. This is particularly so in the types of patient under discussion. The mother is at the end of her labour, is possibly exhausted and has probably accumulated a considerable volume of gastric contents. There is unlikely to be an opportunity to empty the stomach before the start of the procedure, so the hazard of the 'calculated risk' referred to in the previous chapter cannot be avoided. The danger is greatly compounded when general anaesthesia is requested to facilitate delivery of the shoulders or the head in a case of breech presentation, or to enable the obstetrician to deliver a malpresenting second twin. In these circumstances the mother is in the lithotomy position, which causes her basal intra-abdominal pressure to be raised, thereby increasing the danger of vomiting or regurgitation during induction of anaesthesia.

It cannot be too frequently emphasised that general anaesthesia is an unacceptable choice for vaginal delivery with very few and precisely defined exceptions.

Complications immediately after delivery

1. Removal of retained placenta

If a regional block is in progress during delivery of the infant, it will satisfy the anaesthetic requirements for manual removal of the placenta. If the mother did not have an epidural or a spinal, the technique of choice is a spinal block. The analgesia must extend up to the T10 segments, otherwise the patient will experience considerable pain whilst the uterine cavity is being explored and pressure is being externally applied to the fundus of the uterus.

It is not common for excessive blood loss to be a feature of this condition. However, should there be suggestive evidence that the mother is hypovolaemic, blood should rapidly be infused before initiation of the spinal.

If the cervix has contracted to an extent such that the obstetrician has difficulty in inserting his hand into the uterus (usually a consequence of the inadvisable administration of an oxytocic), the mother should be requested to take two breaths of salbutamol from a Ventolin inhaler which will promote relaxation of the uterus. Retraction subsequent to removal of the placenta will be satisfactory if an oxytocin infusion is provided.

As with operative vaginal delivery the choice of a general anaesthetic for manual removal of a placenta should be considered as an admission of inadequacy. The preferred method, if spinal analgesia cannot be made available, is hypoaesthesia as described previously.

2. Acute inversion of the uterus

This condition can present in one of two ways; haemorrhagic shock or neurogenic shock.

In haemorrhagic shock the patient is probably complaining of some pain but it is unlikely to be contributing significantly to her state of shock. The bleeding is venous in origin, and a rapid infusion of appropriately-warmed blood will correct the hypovolaemia sufficiently to relieve the shocked condition of the mother and *allow the safe administration of a general anaesthetic* and subsequent repositioning of the uterus. The technique of anaesthesia should follow the pattern described for caesarean section, but halothane may be required in addition to relax the myometrium. Halothane should be administered in a concentration of 2.0 per cent, and should be withdrawn as soon as the uterus has been repositioned.

Neurogenic shock is due to traction upon the tissues of the pelvic viscera and peritoneum. In this type of acute inversion, blood loss is not a notable feature. Only repositioning of the uterus will reverse the shock, and the operation must be conducted without delay. *The technique is general anaesthesia* and should be as described in the previous paragraph.

Complications after delivery

1. Repair of a third-degree tear

This can be accomplished under an epidural or spinal block, if either has been in progress during the delivery. In other circumstances, a spinal block is the technique of choice. The required spread of analgesia extends no higher than the sacral roots, so that patient should sit upright for 15 seconds after completion of injection of local anaesthetic into the c.s.f.

General anaesthesia is a poor choice for this procedure. If the facilities to provide a spinal are not available, hypoaesthesia plus local infiltration of the wound would be a reasonably acceptable choice.

2. Re-suture of a perineal wound

The remarks made in respect to repair of a third degree tear are equally applicable to this procedure.

3. Post-partum haemorrhage and evacuation of retained products

Occasionally the amount of post-partum blood loss is considerable and haemorrhage appears to be continuing unabated. A regional block would be inadvisable under these circumstances because of the danger of causing profound hypotension and *a general anaesthetic should be administered*. Myometrial relaxation with halothane will not be required, and would indeed be contraindicated whilst a rapid blood transfusion is in progress.

If the blood loss has not been considerable, exploration and evacuation of the uterine cavity may be conducted under a spinal block.

4. Post-partum sterilisation

If the patient has been given an epidural block for labour and delivery, and if it is planned to perform a post-partum sterilisation during the 2–3 days subsequent to delivery, the epidural cannula can be left in place and the operation performed under epidural analgesia. It is advisable to inject a few millilitres of saline through the cannula every 6–8 hours during the interval between delivery and operation, to avoid blockage of the lumen of the cannula with coagulated protein.

Complications of non-obstetric origin

The pregnant patient can be subject to almost any of the ills which might beset a non-pregnant woman of child-bearing age. It would be unwieldy to catalogue here all the common and rare conditions which can influence the anaesthetic management of the obstetric patient but there are some recently published reviews (Fishburne 1979, Mangano 1979, Crawford 1980). Only the more frequently met with conditions will be discussed here.

a. Cardiovascular diseases

1. Acquired heart disease

This is usually of rheumatic origin, and is infrequently symptomatic in industrialised communities. The major challenge to the diminished cardiac reserve occurs during three episodes: (i) at about 30 weeks gestation when cardiac output is at the end of its period of peak height; (ii) throughout the second-stage of labour when the mother in effect indulges in the Valsalva manoeuvre and (iii) the immediate post-partum episode when, due to the abrupt reduction in uterine vascular volume, there is a considerable increase in venous return to the heart.

During the third trimester, the immediate care of the patient falls within the province of the cardiologist but when the patient approaches term, the anaesthetist will become involved. Delivery by elective caesarean section is not specifically indicated for these patients and some would argue is contraindicated in the absence of obstetric indications. The objective is to reduce the burden upon the myocardium during labour and delivery and a continuous lumbar epidural block is admirably fitted to the task. It should be effective such that the urge to bear down in the second-stage is obtunded. As has recently been demonstrated, both the pain of contractions and the bearing-down effort significantly increase maternal oxygen consumption (Hagerdal et al 1983).

In this group those patients who are digitalised may have a fore-shortened labour because of the stimulatory action of digitalis upon the myometrium (Weaver & Pearson 1973). If, under such or allied circumstances, labour progresses so rapidly that the administration of an epidural is not feasible a spinal block should be provided for the second-stage and delivery.

An increasing number of pregnant patients diagnosed as having rheumatic heart disease during childhood or early adulthood will have received a valve replacement (Saka & Marx 1976, Taguchi 1977, Gothard 1978). The obstetric care of these mothers is basically the same but with one significant exception. These patients are usually receiving long-term anti-coagulant prophylaxis. If such is the case, and it is intended to provide the patient with an epidural, I recommend that the coagulation profile should be allowed to return to normal; the epidural is then initiated and anti-coagulant therapy may be recommenced some hours later or shortly after delivery. However, discussion of the care of individual patients with the cardiologist undertaking their long-term supervision is advisable. It is advised that the cannula should not be removed until the coagulation profile has reverted to normal, in case the slight trauma associated with the removal disrupts a vessel wall.

2. Congenital heart disease

Many of the patients who achieve pregnancy having had a congenital defect of the heart, will have had the defect satisfactorily corrected in early or later childhood, and will offer no unusual challenge in their obstetric care. There is, however, an increasing number of others who enter the obstetric list with a severe cardiac lesion. They present a formidable challenge to their medical attendants, including both obstetricians and anaesthetists.

Although this group of patients includes those with a single ventricle (Yuzpe et al 1970) or a simple patent ductus arteriosus, the most frequent challenge is that presented by a patient with pulmonary hypertension and a potential intra-cardiac or extra-cardiac shunt; Eisenmenger's syndrome is the classic example. Such a patient must not be allowed to develop hypotension of any significant degree. She has little respiratory reserve to permit her to bear-down for any appreciable time, and will be placed in great jeopardy if subjected to pulmonary thrombo-emboli. Furthermore, if the patient displays 'cyanotic heart disease', the fetus may have intra-uterine growth retardation and be at considerable risk of dying from intra-uterine asphyxia. *Every effort must be made to avoid delivering these patients by caesarean section,* because of the considerable swings of blood pressure which can occur throughout the entire course of this procedure and because of the increased risk of post-partum pulmonary embolism associated with the operation. The requirements are for a brief labour, free from pain, the avoidance of reflex bearing-down, the provision of supplemental oxygen, and, most important, the provision of informed and watchful supervision. If the delivery suite where the patient is to labour is familiar with the management of lumbar epidural analgesia, this is the best choice (Geicher et al 1979), a fact attested to in several reports (McMurray and Kenny 1982, Midwall et al 1978). *Extreme care must be taken to ensure that the maternal blood pressure does not fall*; if a significant reduction does occur, an alpha-adrenergic stimulating agent such as phenylephrine should be given intravenously. Anti-coagulant prophylaxis should be started immediately after the delivery of the placenta, initially with heparin and an oral agent thereafter.

3. Essential hypertension

The conduct of analgesia and anaesthesia in the obstetric care of these patients does not differ from that detailed for the mother with mild pre-eclampsia.

b. Respiratory disease

It is rare for a patient at term to present with severe respiratory embarrassment due to *active or chronic disease of the respiratory tract*. The exception to this is the growing number of women who survive the childhood hazards of cystic fibrosis (Matson & Capen 1982) and are in danger of developing pulmonary hypertension. If such a patient is encountered a general anaesthetic should be avoided at almost any cost. Delivery by caesarean section, if necessitated, should be conducted under a regional block. For a labouring patient in this category, an epidural is specifically indicated, or a spinal if labour has advanced to the end of the first-stage by the time the mother is admitted to the delivery suite.

1. Asthma

This condition is currently the focus of a debate which is as yet unresolved. One authoritative view is that, if an asthmatic patient comes to section, she should be given a general anaesthetic, because thereby access to the airway is ensured. An opposing opinion is that the stimulation of the upper airways under light anaesthesia can provoke an episode of bronchospasm which might persist until irreversible damage has been caused. Dogmatism is to be avoided and discussion prevail; the matter should be resolved within the coming year or two.

There is reason to suspect that ergometrine administered intravenously to an asthmatic patient can provoke severe bronchospasm.

The topic of respiratory pathology in the pregnant patient has been usefully reviewed by Fishburne (1979).

c. Diseases of the central nervous system

Although these conditions are relatively uncommon among women of child-bearing age, most large obstetric units will book one or two such patients each year. The pattern of progress of most of the well-known neuropathies appears to be little influenced by pregnancy and the choice of analgesia and anaesthesia does not require modification.

Specially, there is no justification for the view that because a mother has, for example, *multiple sclerosis*, she should not be given a regional block. The simple measure of depositing a small volume of local anaesthetic around nerve fibres in the epidural space or within the c.s.f. will exert no influence whatsoever upon the progress of the disease. It is, however, important that the patient appreciates this fact before the block is administered. If she does not, or if she appears to have reservations about the assurance given to her, it is advisable not to administer it, lest protracted and unseemly wrangling (possibly in a court of law) results. Case histories in support of these contentions appearing in the literature (Warren et al 1982, Crawford 1983) in increasing numbers will, it is hoped, help to rebut any maladroit legal quibbling in the future.

A patient with a *cerebro-vascular lesion* is not specifically benefited by being delivered by caesarean section. However, her labour should preferentially be conducted in such a manner as to eliminate all pain and to prevent reflex bearing-down. An epidural is thus the technique of choice. If labour is well advanced when the mother reaches the delivery suite, a spinal block should be administered.

The presence of an *intracranial tumour* is not a contraindication to regional analgesia. In this instance, however, *caudal extra-dural is probably to be preferred over lumbar extra-dural*, because an inadvertent dural tap might lead to coning of the brain-stem.

Migraine, epilepsy and 'burnt-out' c.n.s. infections such as poliomyelitis do not provide contraindications to the administration of regional analgesia.

Pregnancy has a variable and unpredictable effect upon the severity of symptoms due to *myasthenia gravis*. The disease does not provide a specific indication for delivery by caesarean section, but if the operation is to be performed the choice and technique of anaesthesia requires to be little different from that under more normal circumstances. If general anaesthesia is given, customary care will be required in the choice of skeletal muscle relaxation and in observing the patient's recovery from anaesthesia.

A continuous epidural is highly advantageous to the conduct of labour and vaginal delivery of a myasthenic patient, because of the avoidance of fatigue afforded by this technique. The topic is reviewed by Rolbin et al (1978).

d. Renal disease

Although acute and chronic renal disease pose considerable problems in the management of the pregnant patient, their influence upon the pattern of analgesia and anaesthesia is likely to be negligible. The hypertension and proteinuria associated with *chronic nephritis* can mimic or have pre-eclampsia superimposed upon it; the anaesthetist's role in the treatment of a patient in this category is as described with respect to pre-eclampsia alone.

In the care of a patient suffering from the *nephrotic syndrome*, consideration must be given to the severe degree of hypoalbuminaemia which characterises this disease and which is likely to be accentuated during pregnancy. The low level of serum protein will influence the transport pattern of protein-bound drugs, and hence the transplacental migration of these agents. Although there appears to have been little investigation into the matter, it is likely that the rate and extent of transfer of such drugs across the blood-brain barrier will also be considerably modified from normal values as a result of the deficiency of serum proteins. Thus, regional analgesia for either labour or operative delivery is likely to be the technique of choice.

An increasing number of women who have had a *renal transplant* are achieving a pregnancy which is carried to term (Parsons et al 1979). An epidural is an appropriate choice to provide analgesia in labour for these patients. However, I, and probably others, have preferred to administer a general anaesthetic if such a mother requires to be delivered by caesarean section, because the position of the transplanted kidney can complicate the surgical procedure and the routine epidural block might not be extensive enough to afford adequate relief from discomfort and pain.

e. Diseases of the musculo-skeletal system

The only pathological conditions of bone and joint which require comment here are those which involve the lumbo-sacral region. Patients in this category include those with: *prolapsed intervertebral disc; 'sciatica'; chronic low back pain of uncertain origin; spondylolisthesis; ankylosing spondylitis; spina bifida occulta; previously fractured lumbar vertebra or pelvis; spinal fusion; and kyphoscoliosis.*

If such patients are to be delivered by caesarean section the choice of anaesthesia will *not* be governed by the category of the disease, with the exception of a *severe degree of kyphoscoliosis*. This can be associated with respiratory embarrassment especially in a patient close to or at term and there is likely to be considerable compression of the inferior vena cava, which will be abruptly relieved as soon as delivery has been accomplished. These patient should be operated upon in the full lateral position and might benefit from an increased inspiratory positive pressure following delivery, in order to combat pulmonary oedema consequent upon the sudden increase in venous return to the heart. General anaesthesia is, therefore, to be preferred over regional analgesia. Extra vigilance and supervision will be needed during the post-operative care of such patients.

It is extremely important that care be taken in moving mothers with these categories of disease, especially into and out of the lithotomy position, whilst an epidural or a spinal is providing pain relief. Much harm could be caused by incautious manipulation whilst the warning signal of pain is obtunded.

The labour and vaginal delivery of other patients in this general category is preferably conducted under epidural analgesia, tailored to ensure that the bearing-down reflex is abolished. This will reduce considerably the extent of exertion which is otherwise associated with labour and delivery, and thus avoids the imposition of strain and trauma upon the affected structures.

In some circumstances entry into the lumbar epidural space might be impossible; a caudal approach should be sought as an alternative.

f. Endocrine diseases

1. Diabetes

Intervillous blood flow is significantly reduced below the normal range of values in the patient with White Class A diabetes, and the reduction is progressive in more severe grades of the disease (Kaar et al 1980). This characteristic of diabetes undoubtedly contributes significantly to the 5 per cent of 'inescapable' fetal deaths associated with the condition (Drury et al 1977). Thus, as gestation progresses the fetus is in increasing jeopardy even under conditions of strict and efficient control of the diabetic state. Any additional causes of intra-uterine asphyxia and effects from transplacentally-derived depressant drugs during labour and delivery, must be reduced to a minimum. This is of even greater moment if there is co-existing pathology, such as pre-eclampsia or breech presentation.

When there is impoverished placental perfusion, a continuous epidural promotes an increase in intervillous flow, provided that aorto-caval compression is avoided and the systemic blood pressure is not allowed to be unduly lowered. As mentioned in respect to PET, an epidural will not reverse the reduction in intervillous blood flow which is referrable to enlargement of fetal villi (Nylund et al 1982). Attention has also been drawn to the fact that an incrementally increasing infusion acidosis of the fetus is averted by the provision of a satisfactory epidural to a labouring patient.

Finally, the use of epidural analgesia renders the administration of centrally-depressant drugs unnecessary.

For all of these reasons, it is clear that the administration of an epidural is the appropriate choice for the conduct of labour and for delivery by caesarean section of diabetic patients (Brudenell 1978). A spinal should be given if the patient is to be delivered vaginally and there has been no time in which to initiate an epidural. A spinal for caesarean section is not a good choice however, because of the associated high incidence of hypotension with resultant perinatal asphyxia (Datta & Brown 1977).

2. Phaeochromocytoma

This rare condition is mentioned here because it is the cause of a small number of maternal deaths each year, and its presence is difficult to diagnose during pregnancy. Diagnosis depends usually upon the clinicians's alertness that a phaeochromocytoma might be the cause of an unusual pattern of hypertensive episodes. In an excellent review of the subject, Leak et al (1977) noted that *the blood pressure increases when the mother lies down*, possibly because the uterus then presses upon the tumour.

If the diagnosis is made during the final trimester, medical treatment should be provided until term is reached. The mother should be given both alpha and beta-adrenergic blockers, phenoxybenzamine and propanolol being the advised drugs (Leak et al 1977). The patient should be delivered by elective caesarean section and the tumour removed during the same operation. General anaesthesia will be required, in concert with a delicately balanced adjustment of adrenergic stimulators and blockers (Schenker & Granat 1982), although the provision of an epidural has recently been advocated on the grounds that it will block the neurogenic stimulation of the tumour (Stonham & Wakefield 1982).

g. Haematological diseases

1. Disseminated intravascular coagulation

This, and less serious manifestations of coagulation defects, have been referred to in the discussion of pre-eclampsia. Their occurrence in association with other disorders, such as placental abruption and abortion, require no additional expertise from the anaesthetist apart from his general understanding of how to collaborate in the resuscitation and intensive care of these patients.

2. Deep vein thrombosis

If this relatively common complication develops ante-natally it is most likely that anti-coagulant therapy will be started and maintained without interruption until several weeks post-partum. *Under this circumstance, a lumbar epidural block is contra-indicated.* No firm opinion has been documented as to whether or not it is advisable to administer a caudal block. It could reasonably be postulated that the single needle insertion for a caudal would be unlikely to cause damage to an extra-dural vein, while the insertion of a catheter via a Tuohy needle for an epidural could provoke haemorrhage. It is equally unlikely that an epidural vein would be traumatised during the administration of a spinal.

Anti-coagulant therapy can be started within two hours of initiating a lumbar epidural block; it is also acceptable to insert an epidural catheter if anti-coagulant prophylaxis has been temporarily suspended and laboratory investigation confirms that all aspects of the clotting mechanism have reverted to normal.

Deep vein thrombosis (DVT) and its most formidable consequence, pulmonary embolism, occurring post-natally is most frequently related to delivery by caesarean section. The incidence is unknown, but the mortality of the condition is referred to in the triennial issues of Confidential Enquiries into Maternal Deaths in England and Wales. The recorded incidence had been fairly steady until the most recent reports (1973–75 and 1976–78) which showed a marked reduction. My experience has mirrored this on a small scale; from 1968 to 1971 there were two or three patients each year, who developed a DVT after caesarean section. Two suffered a pulmonary embolism, of which one was fatal. Since 1972 no cases of pulmonary embolism have been encountered. The only radical change which was introduced during this period was the use of the wedge to provide a lateral tilt; a practice which has been employed without exception from 1972 onwards. It is reasonable to propose that caval compression at section caused stasis and subsequent thrombosis within the pelvic and leg veins and the 'wedge-tilt' has alleviated such compression.

It could be contended that a continuous epidural provided for labour and delivery diminishes the chance that a mother will develop DVT post-natally because the rate of blood flow through the pelvis and lower limbs is increased as a result of vasodilatation. However, the observation awaits confirmation.

3. Sickle haemoglobinopathies

Only homozygous sickle disease and sickle beta-thalassaemia are likely to pose a threat to the pregnant patient and her fetus (Fiakpui & Moran 1973). Delivery by caesarean section is not specifically indicated, but it is advised that two units of whole blood and two units of washed packed cells be prepared for immediate infusion when the patient is admitted either in labour or for elective section. In order to avoid the production of local venous stasis, with a consequential sickle-cell crisis, very strict supervision of the patient is required to ensure that she is not exposed to aorto-caval compression. If the mother is to labour, an epidural will offer the further advantage of reducing venous stasis. An epidural would be the technique of choice for delivery of such a patient by caesarean section, but if general anaesthesia is provided, pre-oxygenation and the advocated high concentration of oxygen in the inspired mixture should be the rule.

h. Obesity

Obstetricians would be well advised to bear in mind that obesity adds significantly to the risks associated with anaesthesia (Marx & Hodgkinson 1980). It is often very difficult to maintain a patent airway on an obese patient, and endotracheal intubation is rendered more difficult because of the thick, frequently short, neck. The bulk of the patient's soft tissues, including the breasts, tends to reduce the efficiency of ventilation in the post-anaesthetic recovery period. The location of a vein suitable for setting up an infusion can also be a lengthy procedure in these patients.

There is evidence that the incidence of PET is considerably higher among obese subjects than among those of normal weight, and maternal mortality is correlated directly with the weight of the mother. Hodgkinson & Husain (1980) have reported that the spread of a given volume of local anaesthetic within the epidural space is more extensive in the more obese subjects.

Although gross obesity is met with less frequently in the U.K. than in the U.S.A. examples of less extreme forms are not uncommon in obstetric practice. For such patients, caution and advance preparation are advisable in order to reduce the necessity of hurried intervention. If delivery by caesarean section is likely to be required, it is better performed electively and at relative leisure rather than in haste. Experienced anaesthetic aid will be required. There is likely to be considerable difficulty in locating and entering the epidural space of an obese patient. Should it appear likely that she will require an epidural, it should, if possible, be initiated early in labour. As Hodgkinson & Husain (1981) have reported, the extent of spread of solution injected into the epidural space tends to be relatively increased in association with obesity.

i. Miscellaenous

Certain other categories of non-obstetric pathology are worthy of mention in the context of the present discussion.

Von Willebrand's disease affords another example of the use to which the Cardiff Palliator can be put. An epidural is contra-indicated for mothers with this condition, and intramuscular injections are inadvisable.

Although death due to haemorrhage is characteristic of type IV Ehlers-Danlos syndrome, this is due to defects of connective tissue and not to a coagulation defect. An epidural is not contra-indicated for labouring mothers with this condition, but, because of their tendency to excessive blood loss from either a perineal laceration or an atonic uterus, they must remain under intensive observation for several days postpartum (Abouleish 1980). An epidural block is not contra-indicated for the relief of pain of a labouring patient with myotonia dystrophica who, if she has carried her pregnancy to the third trimester, is likely to go into premature labour (Webb et al 1978). The labour might be brief or, because of inco-ordinate uterine activity, very prolonged, and inefficient uterine retraction is a likely complication to be anticipated.

Genital herpes does not pose a contra-indication to regional analgesia, whether for caesarean section or vaginal delivery. Viraemia is most unlikely to be present at the time that these mothers are ready to be delivered.

On general grounds it appears to be likely that an epidural for labour will be of benefit particularly in the labour of a mother whose pregnancy has advanced beyond 42 weeks. In such a situation there is an increased likelihood of intrapartum fetal asphyxia or death (Devoe & Sholl 1983), which is, in part at least, probably due to an inefficiency of intervillous blood flow.

REFERENCES

Abouleish E 1980 Obstetric anaesthesia and Ehlers-Danlos syndrome. British Journal of Anaesthesia 52: 1283

Berkowitz R L 1980 Anti-hypertensive drugs in the pregnant patient. Obstetric & Gynecological Reviews 35: 191

Birmingham Eclampsia Study Group 1971 Intravascular coagulation & abnormal lung scans in pre-eclampsia. Lancet 2: 889

Breeson A J, Kovacs G T, Pickles B G, Hill J G 1978 Extradural analgesia — the preferred method of analgesia for vaginal breech delivery. British Journal of Anaesthesia 50: 1227

Brudenell J M 1978 Delivering the baby of the diabetic mother. In: Diabetes in pregnancy: a symposium. Journal of the Royal Society of Medicine 71: 207

Crawford J S 1958a Anaesthesia for obstetrics: recent advances. British Medical Bulletin 14: 34

Crawford J S 1958b Obstetric anaesthesia. Practitioners 181: 232

Crawford J S 1974 An appraisal of lumbar epidural blockade in patients with a singleton fetus presenting by the breech. Journal of Obstetrics & Gynaecology of the British Commonwealth 81: 867

Crawford J S 1975 An appraisal of lumbar epidural blockade in labour in patients with multiple pregnancy. British Journal of Obstetrics & Gynaecology 118: 700

Crawford J S 1976 The epidural sieve & MBC (minimum blocking concentration): an hypothesis. Anaesthesia 31: 1227

Crawford J S 1979 Experience with spinal analgesia in a British obstetric unit. British Journal of Anaesthesia 51: 531

Crawford J S 1980 Medical Diseases in pregnancy In: Vickers M D Medicine for Anaesthetists, 2nd edn. Blackwell, Oxford

Crawford J S 1983 Epidural analgesia for patients with chronic neurological disease. Anesthesia & Analgesia 62: 617

Datta S, Brown W U 1977 Acid-base status in diabetic mothers and their infants following general or spinal anesthesia for cesarean section. Anesthesiology 47: 272

De Crespigny L J C, Pepperell R J 1979 Perinatal mortality and morbidity in breech presentation. Obstetrics & Gynecology 53: 141

Devoe L D, Sholl J S 1983 Postdates pregnancy. Journal of Reproductive Medicine 28: 576

Drury M I, Greene A T, Stronge J M 1977 Pregnancy complicated by clinical diabetes mellitus. Obstetrics & Gynecology 49: 519

Fiakpui E Z, Moran E M 1973 Pregnancy in sickle hemoglobinopathies. Journal of Reproductive Medicine 11: 28

Fishburne J 1979 Physiology & disease of the respiratory system in pregnancy. Journal of Reproductive Medicine 22: 177

Gleicher N, Midwall J, Hochberger D, Jaggin H 1979 Eisenmenger's Syndrome & pregnancy. Obstetric & Gynecologic Survey 34: 721

Gothard J W W 1978 Heart disease in pregnancy. Anaesthesia 33: 523

Gullestad S, Sagan N 1977 Epidural block in twin labour & delivery. Acta anaesthesiologica scandinavica 21: 504

Hagerdal M, Morgan C W, Sumner A E, Gutsche B B 1983 Minute ventilation and oxygen consumption during labor with epidural analgesia. Anesthesiology 59: 425

Harper N J N, Thomson J, Brayshaw S A 1983 Experience with self-administered pethidine with special reference to the general practitioner obstetric unit. Anaesthesia 38: 52

Henshall W R 1979 Differences in albumin distribution & dynamics between toxaemic & non-toxaemic pregnant women. British Journal of Obstetrics & Gynaecology 86: 463

Hodgkinson R, Husain F J 1980 Obesity & the cephalad spread of analgesia following epidural administration of bupivacaine for cesarean section. Current Researches in Anesthesia & Analgesia 59: 89

Hodgkinson R, Husain F J 1981 Obesity, gravity and spread of epidural anesthesia. Anesthesia and Analgesia 60: 421

Hutchins C J 1980 Spinal analgesia for instrumental delivery. Anaesthesia 35: 376

James F M, Crawford J S, Davies P, Naiem H 1977 Lumbar epidural analgesia for labour & delivery of twins. American Journal of Obstetrics & Gynecology 127: 176

Jarvis G J, Whitefield M F 1981 Epidural analgesia and the delivery of twins. Journal of Obstetrics and Gynaecology 2: 90

Jaschevatzky O E, Shalit A, Levy Y, Grunstein S 1977 Epidural analgesia during labour in twin pregnancy. British Journal of Obstetrics & Gynaecology 84: 327

Jouppila R, Jouppila P, Hollmen A, Koivula A 1979 Epidural analgesia & placental blood flow during labour in pregnancies complicated by hypertension. British Journal of Obstetrics & Gynaecology 86: 969

Joyce T H, Debnath K S, Baker E A 1979 Pre-eclampsia — relationship of c.v.p. and epidural analgesia. Anesthesiology 51: S297

Kaar K, Jouppila P, Kuikka J, Luotola H, Toivanen J, Rekonen A 1980 Intervillous blood flow in normal and uncomplicated late pregnancy measured by means of an intravenous ^{133}Xe method. Acta obstetricia gynecologica scandinavica 59: 7

Leak D, Carroll J J, Robinson D C, Ashworth E J 1977 Management of phaeochromocytoma during pregnancy. Canadian Medical Association Journal 116: 371

McMurray T J, Kenny N T 1982 Extradural anaesthesia in parturients with severe cardiovascular disease. Anaesthesia 37: 442

Mangano D T 1979 Anesthesia for the pregnant cardiac patient. In: Shnider S M, Levinson G. (eds) Anesthesia for obstetrics, William & Wilkins, Baltimore/London.

Martin C B, McGaughey M S, Kaiser I H, Donner M W, Ramsey E M 1964 Intermittent functioning of the retroplacental arteries. American Journal of Obstetrics & Gynecology 90: 819

Marx G F, Hodgkinson R 1980 Special considerations in complications of pregnancy In: Marx G F, Bassell G M (eds) Obstetric analgesia & anesthesia. Excerpta medica, Amsterdam/Oxford/New York

Matson J A, Capen C V 1982 Pregnancy in the cystic fibrosis patient. Journal of Reproductive Medicine 27: 373

Midwall J, Jaffin J, Herman M V, Kupersmith J 1978 Shunt flow & pulmonary hemodynamics during labour & delivery in Eisenmenger's syndrome. American Journal of Cardiology 42: 299

Moir D D, Victor-Rodrigues L, Willocks J 1972 Epidural analgesia during labour in patients with pre-eclampsia. Journal of Obstetrics & Gynaecology of the British Commonwealth 79: 465

Nylund L, Lunell N O, Lewander R, Persson B, Sarby B 1982 Uteroplacental blood flow in diabetic pregnancy. American Journal of Obstetrics and Gynecology 144: 298

Parsons V, Bewick M, Elias J, Snowden S A, Weston M J, Rodeck C H 1979 Pregnancy following renal transplantation. Journal of the Royal Society of Medicine 72: 815

Power G G, Longo L D, Wagner H N, Kuhle D E, Forster R E 1967 Uneven distribution of maternal & fetal placental blood flow, as demonstrated using macroaggregates, and its response to hypoxia. Journal of Clinical Investigation 46: 2053

Rolbin S H, Levinson G, Shnider S M, Wright R G 1978 Anesthetic considerations for myasthenia gravis & pregnancy. Current Researches in Anesthesia & Analgesia 57: 441

Saka D M, Marx G F 1976 Management of a parturient with cardiac valve prosthesis. Current Researches in Anestheseia & Analgesia 55: 214

Schenker J E, Granat M 1982 Phaeochromocytoma and pregnancy: an updated appraisal. Australia and New Zealand Journal of Obstetrics and Gynaecology 22: 1

Scudamore J H, Yates M J 1966 Pudendal block: a misnomer? Lancet 1: 23

Seager S J, Macdonald R 1980 Laryngeal oedema & pre-eclampsia. Anaesthesia 35: 360

Sehgal N N, Hitt J R 1980 Plasma volume expansion in the treatment of pre-eclampsia. American Journal of Obstetrics and Gynecology 138: 165

Snyder S W, Wheeler A S, James F M 1979 Use of nitroglycerine to control severe hypertension of pregnancy during cesarean section. Anesthesiology 51: 563

Stonham J, Wakefield C 1982 Phaeochromocytoma in pregnancy. Anaesthesia 38: 654

Taguchi K 1977 Pregnancy in patients with prosthetic heart valve. Surgery Gynecology & Obstetrics 145: 206

Talledo E O, Chesley L C, Zuspan F P 1968 Renin-angiotensin system in normal & toxemic pregnancies II. American Journal of Obstetrics & Gynecology 100: 218

Templeton A A, Kelman G R 1977 Arterial blood gases in pre-eclampsia. British Journal of Obstetrics & Gynaecology 84: 290

Warren T M, Datta S, Ostheimer G W 1982 Lumbar epidural analgesia in a patient with multiple sclerosis. Anesthesia and Analgesia 61: 1022

Weaver J B, Pearson J F 1973 Influence of digitalis on time of onset & duration of labour in women with cardiac disease. British Medical Journal 3: 519

Webb D, Muir I, Faulkner J, Johnson G 1978 Myotonia dystrophica: obstetric complications. American Journal of Obstetrics and Gynecology 132: 265

Weeks A R L, Cheridjian V E, Mwanje D K 1977 Lumbar epidural analgesia in labour in twin pregnancy. British Medical Journal 2: 730

Whitney D J 1966 Manual removal of the placenta using intravenous analgesia. Journal of Obstetrics & Gynaecology of the British Commonwealth 73: 988

Yuzpe A A, Johnson F L, Robinson J G 1970 Successful pregnancy in a patient with single ventricle & other congenital cardiac anomalies. Canadian Medical Association Journal 103: 1073

Index

166

Index